A JOURNAL FOR <u>NON</u> JOURNALERS

GIVE YOURSELF SELFLOVE

Joelle Rabow Maletis. MAED. MA. LMFT

Publishing: Talk+Tell
Cover art: Mattea Henderson

Distribution by KDP Amazon and Ingram Spark (P.O.D.)
Printed in the United States of America and Canada

Title: Give Yourself SelfLove
Names: Joelle Rabow Maletis
Website: www.joellerabowmaletis.com

Paperback ISBN: 978-1-7357013-3-2
Hardcover ISBN: 978-1-7357013-2-5
E-book ISBN: 978-1-7357013-4-9

Book description: A workbook that teaches self-love and helps people learn that loving themselves is the first step to a life of happiness and fulfillment.

Dedication

Thank you to everyone who helped me on this journey. From the bottom of my heart, I appreciate all the work everyone has done.Marco, you inspire me with your talent and empathy; I am a better mother, clinician, and human because of you. Alexa, your wisdom, strength and devotion are beyond your years; you continue to move me forward to become the best version of all of me every day. Michael, your love is fuel.

Hello Friends!

Why does self-care seem so daunting? It's hard to identify what self-care actually is and how to implement it when it should be easy, which we often say to ourselves. I think this is where we go sideways- it's not easy - there's no should about it. Let's look at it from creating micro-self care: little changes we can make for ourselves, every day, that help us rejuvenate while becoming more resilient. As a licensed marriage and family therapist, trauma-expert, TED Talk speaker, and world renowned trauma expert, I've created this workbook to help you create the life YOU LOVE! Here's my top 5 Micro Self Care Favs: one, clean up my desk and organize; two, add fresh fruit in my water and drink more of it (try lime, lemon, or blueberry); three, listen to a fun playlist of my favorite tunes (can you say Lizzo?); four, send a silly joke/meme to my BFFs; and five, practice kindness towards myself by implementing 1-4 as well as practicing kindness towards others. When all else fails, I enjoy sipping a refreshing, decaf iced drink outside in nature. It always makes me feel better. My challenge to you for the next 31 days: use the book (based on empirically-researched and psycho-educational therapeutic skills) to help you create new micro-self care habits, change your self-shoulding, and move into a new way of being present; by manifesting a better version of you, you continue to grow into the amazing person YOU already are! Celebrate your wins and embrace your failures; tomorrow you get to start again on your self love journey!

Be well,

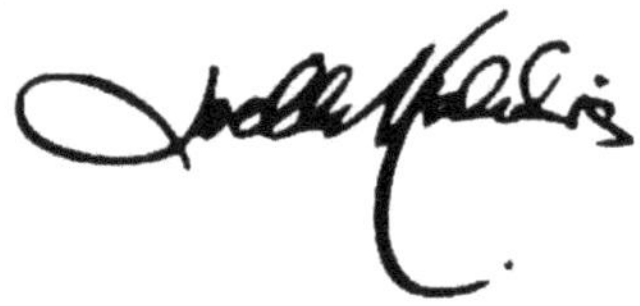

Table of Contents
PERSONAL ACTION PLAN

Introduction

The Give Yourself Self Love: A Journal for Non-Journalers will help you work towards your best self by allowing you to: IDENTIFY, CHALLENGE and REPLACE your beliefs about you - getting to GROW yourself through personal exploration. Over the next 31 days, you'll be able to move from surviving to THRIVING! Your personal growth process is your journey of developing and improving yourself in various areas of life; such as emotionally, intellectually, physically, and spiritually. Making a commitment to your personal growth means cultivating your self-love through practicing self-awareness, self-discovery, and self-improvement skills, having a willingness to learn and expanding a growth mindset. Ultimately, finding fulfillment and joy in the person you are every day by showing up and making a commitment to loving yourself for you!

The IDENTIFY, CHALLENGE and REPLACE process is founded in extensive research steeped in empirically-based psychotherapeutic methodology that is peer-reviewed! Through skills and self-reflection prompts, you'll be able to clearly identify issues that are holding you back from living your BEST (not perfect) self. You will learn to challenge negative beliefs, thoughts, feelings and responses then replace your negative patterns with new skills in just 31 days. And, it works! Over 15 years and thousands of clients, this methodology has been proven to increase your overall joy.

Give Yourself Self Love: A Journal for Non-Journalers allows you to create, develop, manage, maintain and inspire your self-love! Your Personal growth journey and action plan is an ongoing process that requires practice, patience, dedication, and a willingness to learn - even just spending 5 minutes every day - you'll increase your happiness.

By breaking down your experiences into small digestible parts, you can begin to understand yourself more deeply. The beginning of this journey is exciting and may be a bit terrifying all at the same time! This is normal; the human brain has the capacity to feel both excited and terrified simultaneously. Remember that there's no "right way" to take good care of yourself. Your journey is about your individual process that works best for you.

Believe in yourself; understand that your experience will be a valuable and meaningful one as you're working towards positive change. When using the IDENTIFY, CHALLENGE and REPLACE framework, you can improve your self-love and navigate a life that is more meaningful to you!

Here are the steps for taking care of yourself during your Give Yourself Self Love: A Journal for Non-Journalers exploration:

1. Safety and stabilization:

The first step to better self-care is to establish a sense of safety and stability.

2. Emotional processing:

It is essential to begin working through the emotions, behaviors and memories that bring you difficulty.

3. Cognitive restructuring:

By challenging negative thoughts and beliefs about ourselves and the world, we can learn to develop a more positive and joyful outlook.

4. Building resilience:

Through developing skills and strategies to manage stressors and cope with difficulties we can increase our strength in dealing with adversity.

5. Reintegration:

The final step is to reintegrate back into daily life by implementing your new skills into your daily life and living.

Although Changing behavior can feel like a complex and challenging process, there are several strategies that can be helpful in facilitating positive behavior modification. Remember even just 5 minutes daily will yield positive experiences and a noticeable change. When using the IDENTIFY, CHALLENGE and REPLACE framework, remember to follow these guidelines:

1. Setting clear SMART goals:

Identify specific, measurable goals that you want to achieve, and create a plan of action for reaching those goals.

2. Identifying triggers:

Identify the situations or environmental factors that trigger the behavior you want to change, and develop strategies for managing those triggers.

3. Practicing self-awareness:

Pay attention to your thoughts, feelings, and behaviors, and try to identify patterns or habits that may be contributing to the behavior you want to change.

4. Building new habits:

Replace the old behavior with a new, healthier habit by practicing it consistently over time. This can help to reinforce the new behavior and make it a natural part of your routine. A habit is a behavior or pattern of behavior that is repeated regularly and tends to occur subconsciously, without much conscious thought or effort.

5. Seeking support:

Seek out support from friends, family, or a mental health professional who can provide encouragement, accountability, and guidance as you work to change your behavior.

6. Positive reinforcement:
Uses rewards or incentives to reinforce or encourage a particular behavior you're wanting to change. It involves providing a desirable consequence or reward immediately following a behavior, in order to increase the likelihood that the behavior will be repeated in the future.

7. Being Patient:
Remember practice makes almost perfect; your goal is your best-not-perfect-self. It is important to remember that changing behavior takes time and effort, and setbacks are a normal part of the process.

8. Please be mindful:
Emotional growth work often involves stepping out of one's comfort zone and taking risks in order to achieve personal goals and aspirations. If you find that this process is too difficult or you're struggling, please stop and seek professional therapeutic help immediately. This may involve working with a mental health professional to develop coping strategies to manage symptoms, and creating a safe and supportive environment.

9. Self-love
Refers to the practice of caring for, accepting, and valuing oneself. It involves developing a positive and nurturing relationship with oneself, recognizing one's worth, and prioritizing one's own well-being. Self-love encompasses self-compassion, self-acceptance, and maintaining healthy boundaries. It is an essential aspect of personal growth, contributing to improved mental, emotional, and physical well-being."

By developing your personal growth action plan, you'll learn how to overcome challenges, develop new skills, and discover a new sense of self through this empirically-based skills workbook facilitating change. Using Give Yourself Self Love: A Journal for Non-Journalers, you will develop a growth mindset while expanding your knowledge, developing new self-love skills, assisting your self-love discovery, and thriving instead of surviving!

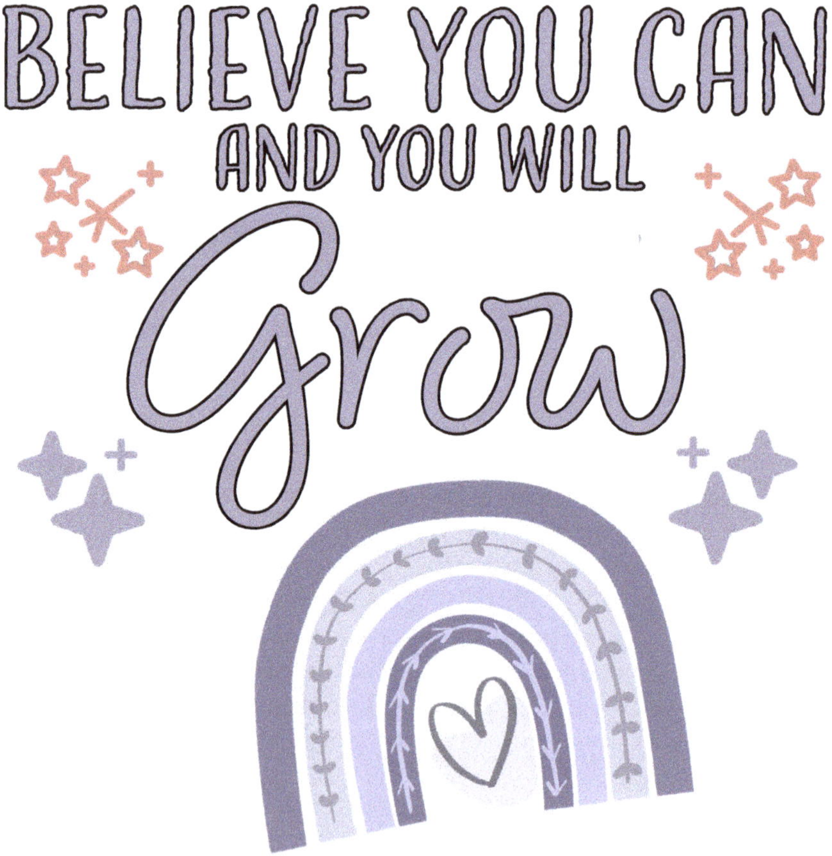

How You Can Work Towards Growth Using This Workbook

Create a Personal Action Plan

Develop your Personal Action Plan by making one small change every day. The skills in this book are crafted based on using empirically-based psychological treatment models to help you make the changes you desire. Go at your own pace; take as much or as little time as you need. All the questions can be done as thought exercises if you'd rather "think" than "write". You can do the whole workbook as fast as you want - do it over and over for 31 days and you'll notice a positive change - commit to YOU for 31 days and see what you accomplish. There is no way to fail at this... if you find you don't have time then put the workbook down for a while until you do have time. The control is in your hands- the process will be exactly what you need in this moment right now! I BELIEVE IN YOU! Please believe in YOU TOO!

day
1

Smart Goals

Goals are the desired outcomes or achievements that a person wants to attain. They help provide direction and motivation, which can be either short-term or long-term in nature. Setting goals can be helpful in personal and professional development, by clarifying what is important as well as needed to be accomplished. (p.333)

YOU ARE ALLOWED TO BE SENSITIVE.

YOU ARE ALLOWED TO PUT YOURSELF FIRST.

YOU ARE ALLOWED TO OUTGROW PEOPLE.

YOU ARE ALLOWED TO TAKE UP SPACE.

YOU ARE ALLOWED TO FEEL TIRED.

YOU ARE ALLOWED TO LOVE WHO YOU WANT.

YOU ARE ALLOWED TO GRIEVE.

YOU ARE ALLOWED TO BE SCARED.

YOU ARE ALLOWED TO BE DIFFERENT.

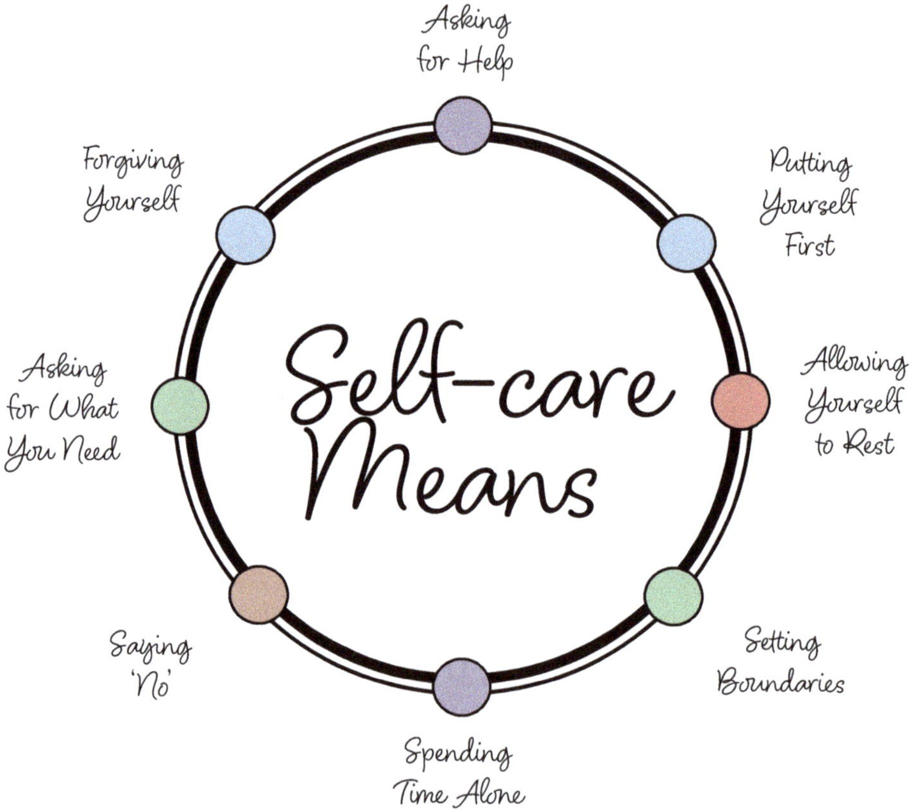
Self-care Means
Asking for Help
Putting Yourself First
Allowing Yourself to Rest
Setting Boundaries
Spending Time Alone
Saying 'No'
Asking for What You Need
Forgiving Yourself

Self-care Jar

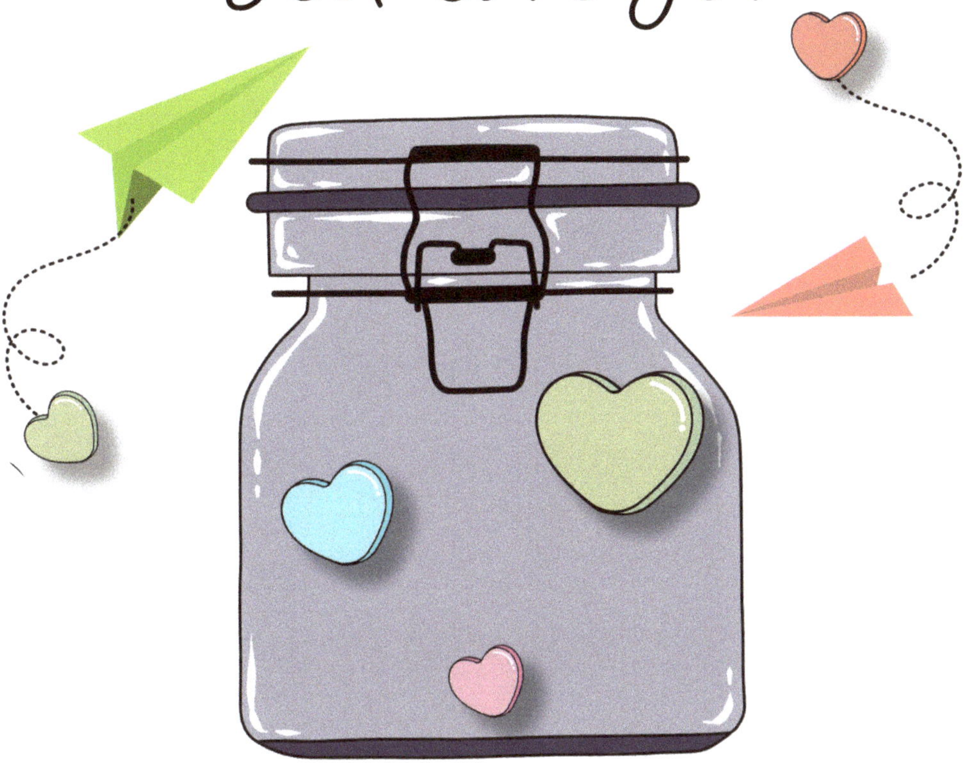

1. Get an empty jar.

2. Write down your favorite micro self-care activities on strips of paper. Then put them inside the jar.

3. In moments of low mood, high stress, or exhaustion, select a strip of paper and proceed to carry out the micro self-care activity written on it.

Hello Change:

MOVE FROM SURVIVING TO THRIVING

Growing

Openness

Alignment

Living

Surrender

Fears get in our way and stop us from achieving our **GOALS**! Change one small thing each day, and create a new habit!

My Bucket List

Things I want to do

Make your list below

S.M.A.R.T. Goals

S. **Specific**
You have clearly defined actions you will be following to reach your goals.

M. **Measurable**
There are ways that you can measure your progress and success over time.

A. **Attainable**
The goal is attainable and realistic for you based on current habits.

R. **Relevant**
It's important to you that you achieve this based on your values and emotions.

T. **Time-bound**
You can measure your success over a set period of time.

S.M.A.R.T. Goals

For More Self-Love

Write them down below.

S. Specific

M. Measurable

A. Attainable

R. Relevant

T. Time-bound

day 2

Self-Love Needs

Self-love is the process that enables us to appreciate and accept ourselves for who we are, flaws and all. When we love ourselves, we are better equipped to handle life's challenges, set healthy boundaries, have fulfilling relationships, pursue our goals and live our dreams (p.335)

My Pyramid of Basic Self-Love Needs

What do you need every day to LOVE YOURSELF?

I need ....
1-3 days a week

I need ....
2-5 days a week

I need ....
4-6 days a week

I need ....
5-7 days a week

I need ....
All day, every day

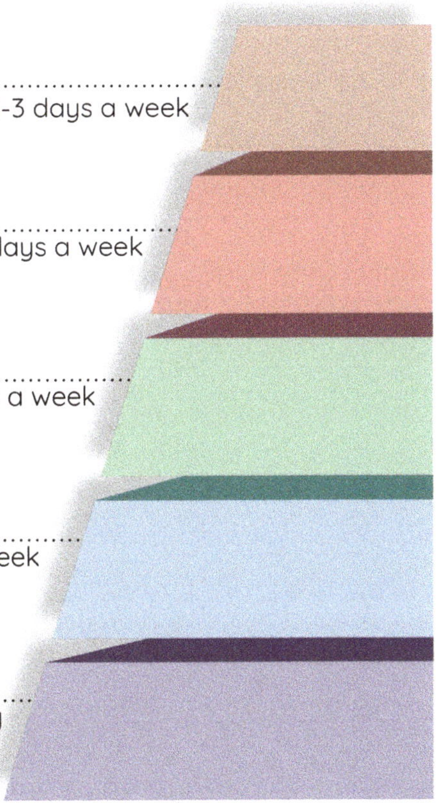

What is Happening

Inside Your Brain. . .

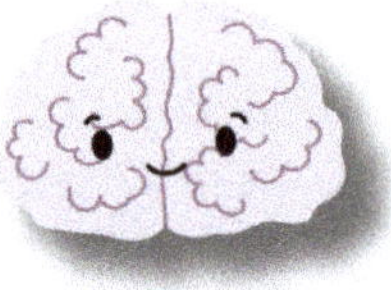

Sensory Cortex

- Sensations
- Movement
- Planning

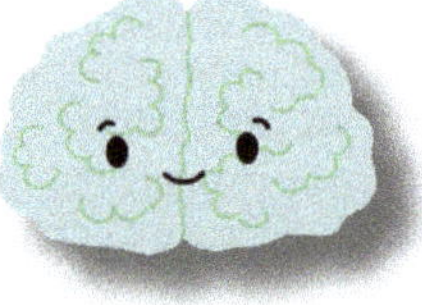

Pre-frontal Cortex

- Logic
- Rational thought
- Decision making

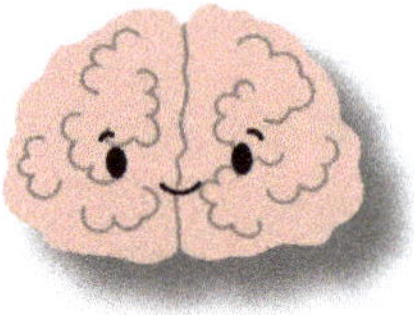

Amygdala

- Threat detection (fight, flight and freeze)

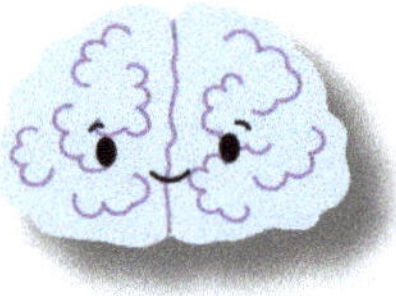

Hypothalamus

- Emotional regulation
- Sleep & wake cycle
- Appetite/hunger

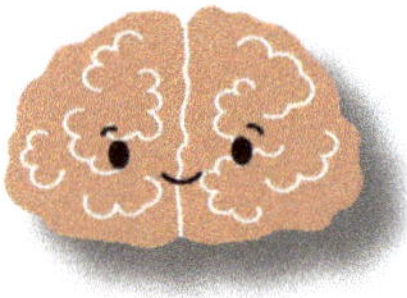

Hippocampus

- Learning
- Memory

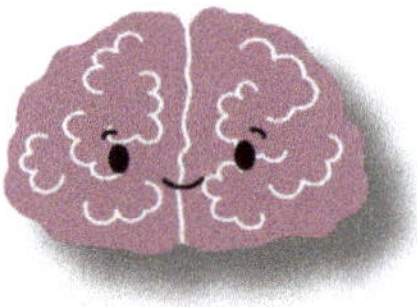

Brain Stem

- Breathing
- Heart rate
- Blood Circulation

Do you ever wonder what is actually going on in your brain? Here is a short synopsis of what is happening!

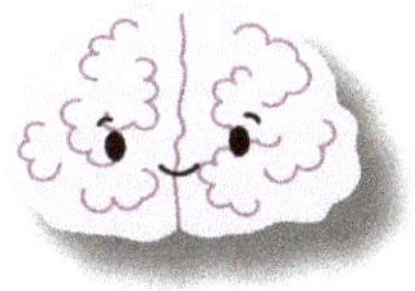

The **sensory cortex** is controlling your sensations, movement, and planning.

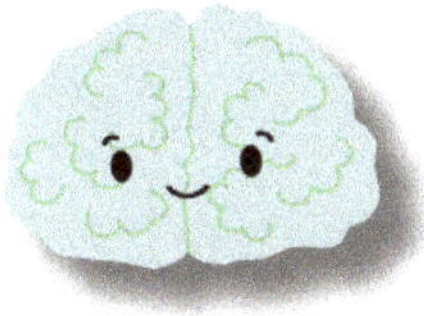

The **prefrontal cortex** is controlling logic, rational thoughts, decisions and planning.

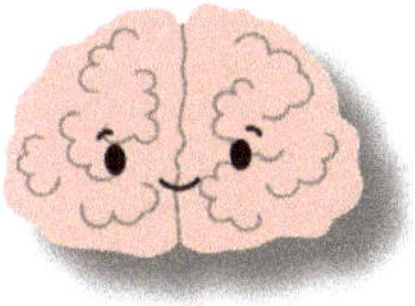

The **amygdala** is controlling threat detection and facilitates the fight, flight and freeze responses.

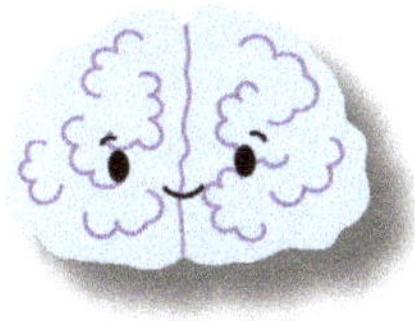

The **hypothalamus** is controlling your emotional regulation, sleep, appetite, sex drive, and temperature.

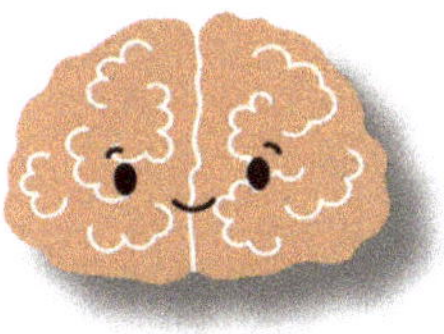

The **hippocampus** controls memory and learning.

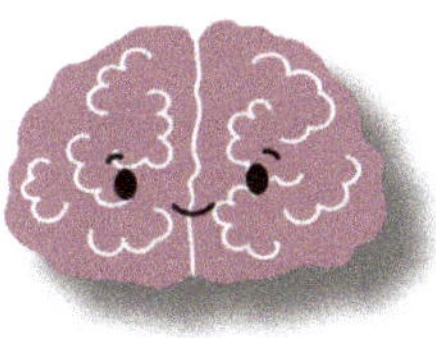

Last but not least, the brainstem controls breathing, swallowing, heart rate, and blood circulation.

Mental Health Exercises

Ways to Care For Yourself

Check off a "to-do"

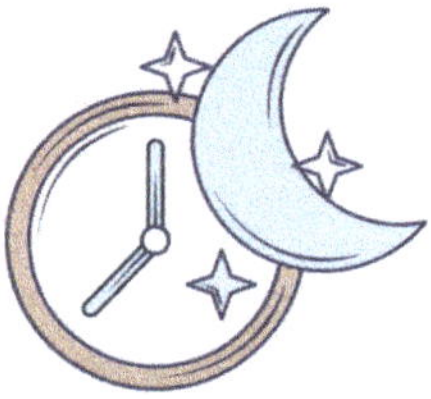

Go to bed 30 minutes early

Say "no" to something

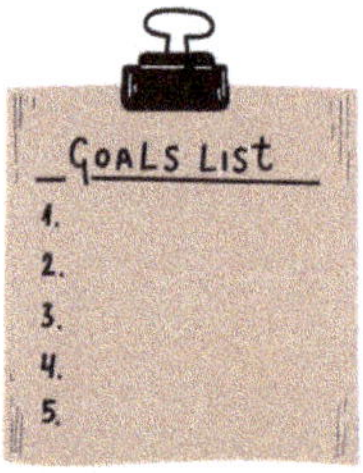

Set mini goals

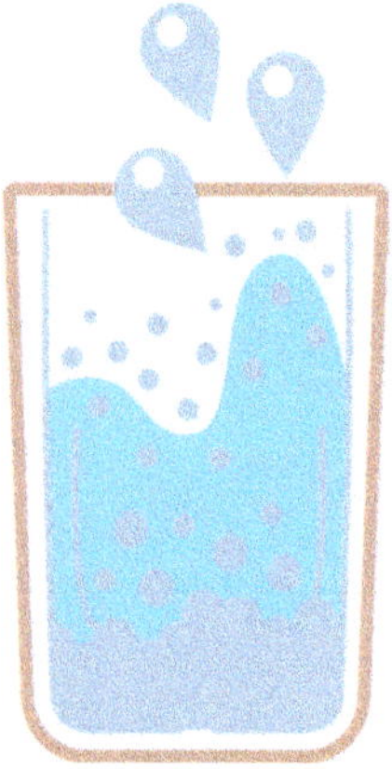

Drink extra water

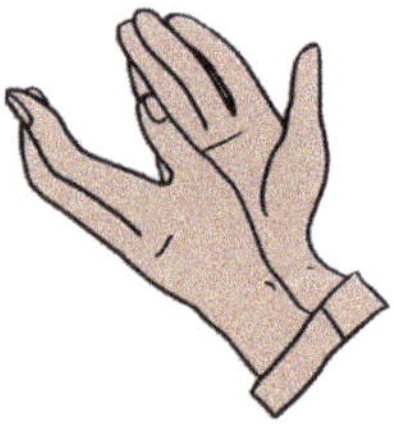

Compliment someone and yourself

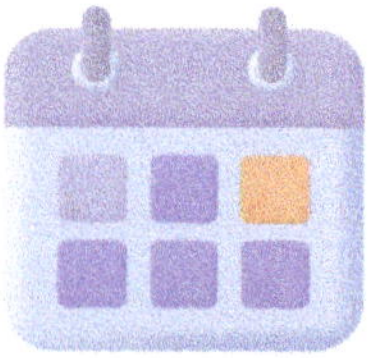

Make time for a task you've been putting off

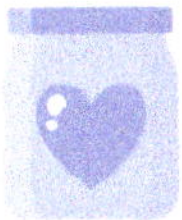

Mental health exercises are an important part of self-care that can help improve overall well-being and help us cope with stress, negative mental health.

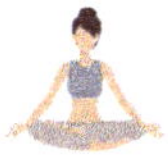

These exercises can include a variety of practices such as goal setting, positive affirmations, increasing sleep, making time for self care, and setting boundaries.

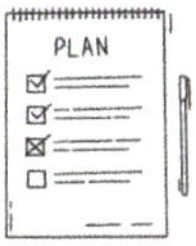

They can be done at home, at work or on the go, and can be as simple as taking a few minutes each day to focus on your breath and clear your mind, or as structured as working with a therapist to develop a specific treatment plan.

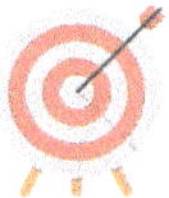

It's important to find the right exercises that work for you and to make them a regular part of your routine.

By prioritizing your mental health and taking care of yourself, you can improve your mood, reduce stress, and increase your overall sense of well-being.

What will you make a priority today?

This Week's Mantras

Try one every night before you head to bed!

Today I was brave!

Today I faced my fears!

Today I was present!

Today I was my best self!

Today I was amazing!

Today I worked hard!

It's Ok

ALLOW YOURSELF TO...

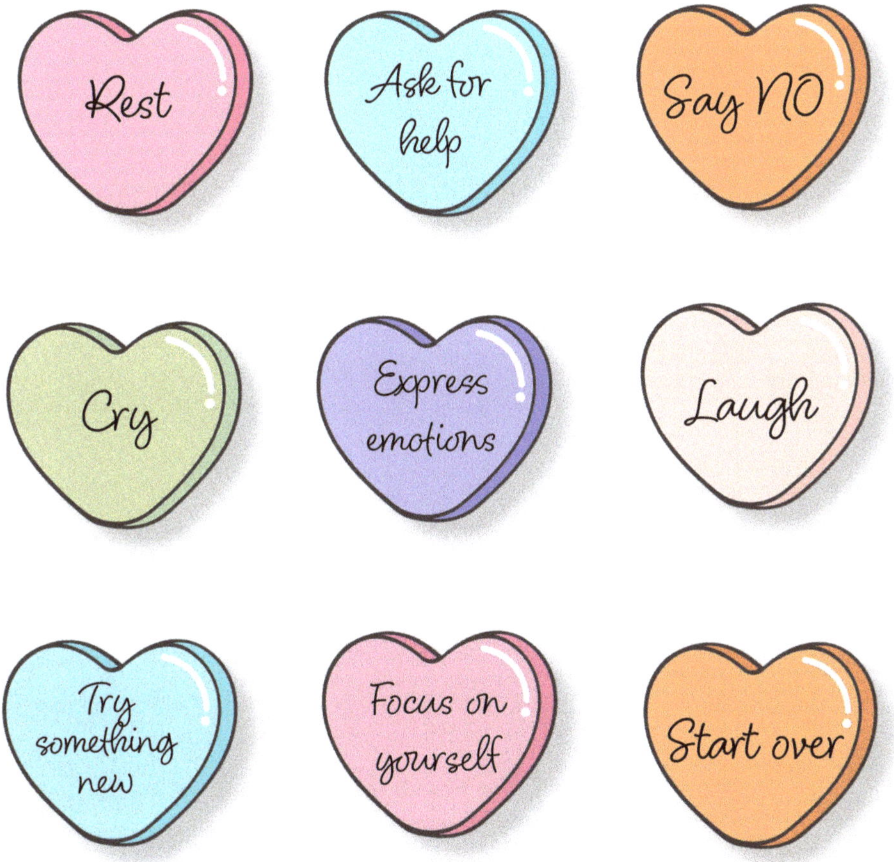

day 3

Self-Esteem Boost

Self-esteem refers to an individual's overall subjective evaluation of their worth, value, and adequacy as a person; to the degree at which they see themselves as capable, lovable, and deserving of respect and dignity. Self-esteem can be influenced by a range of factors, including one's upbringing, experiences, achievements, and social relationships. (p.335)

How Are You Feeling Today?

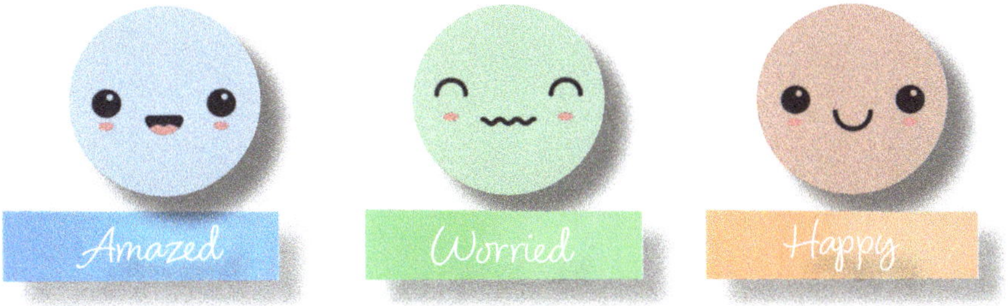

Why do you feel this way? Write your answer below!

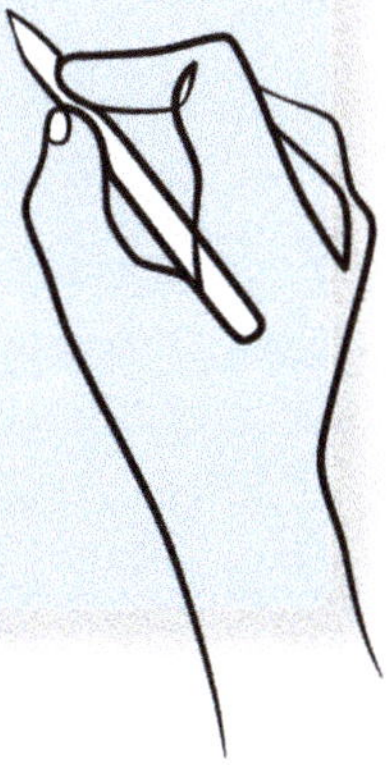

Ways to Boost Self-Esteem

Ways to Care For Yourself

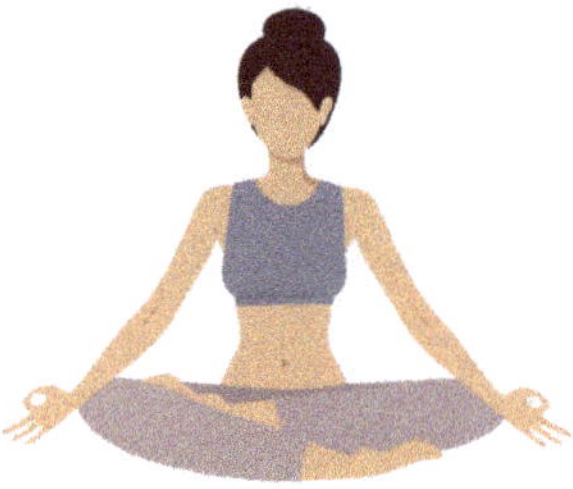

Practice meditation and mindfulness

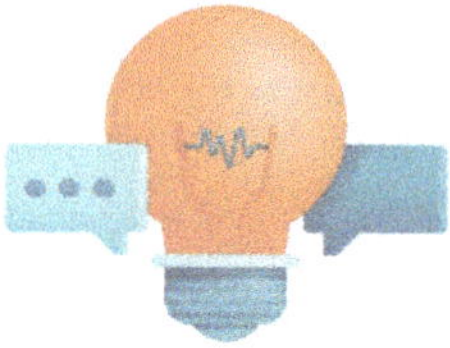

Challenge your inner dialogue

Surround yourself with positive people

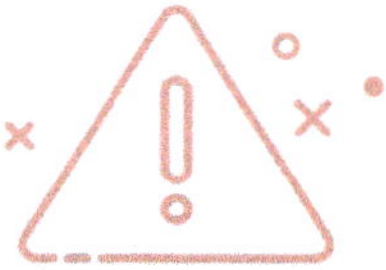

Stop apologizing for things that aren't your fault

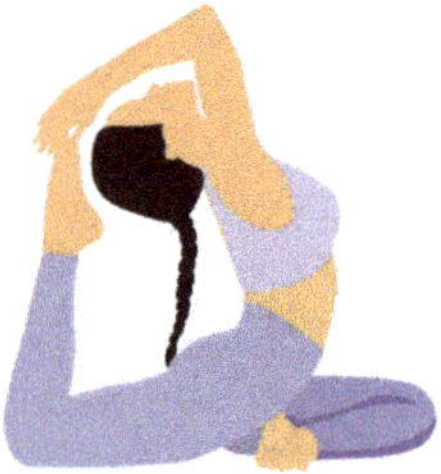

Prioritize exercise that feels good for your body

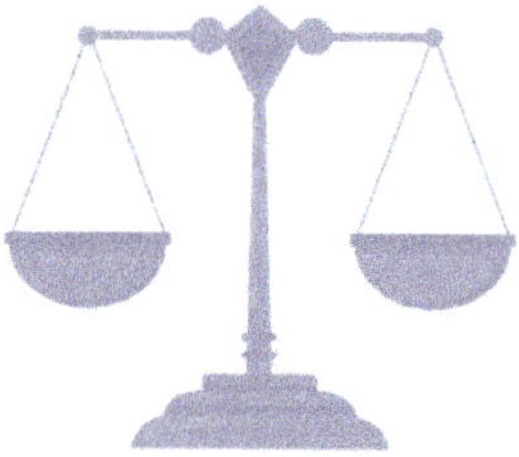

Notice, and limit comparisons to others

I want to improve my self-esteem because:

Practicing mindfulness or meditation can be a great way to begin your day. Both of them can help to improve mood, wellbeing, and increase positive emotions.

It is also helpful to challenge your negative thoughts about yourself by asking, "How do I know this is true?" and "What evidence do I have to support these negative thoughts?"

By challenging your harsh inner critic, you can learn to accept your faults and develop healthier thinking habits.

It's also time to stop over-apologizing! Try to avoid saying "sorry" to others too often and believe in yourself!

Finally, limit your comparisons to others. Rather than focusing on the things others have, try recognizing all the things you have and the qualities you cherish in yourself.

Micro Self-Care Do More Lists:

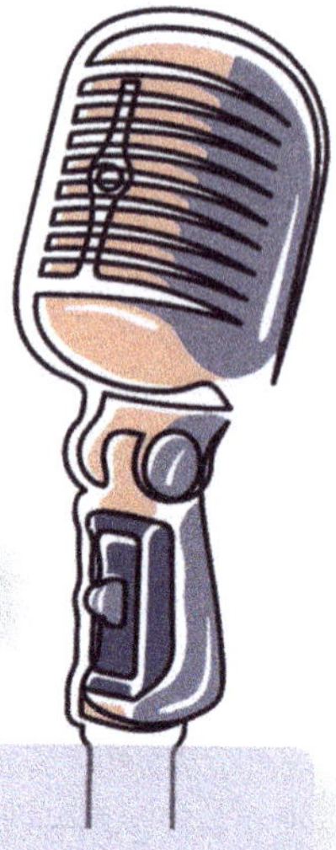

What gives me comfort?

Micro Self-Care Do More Lists:

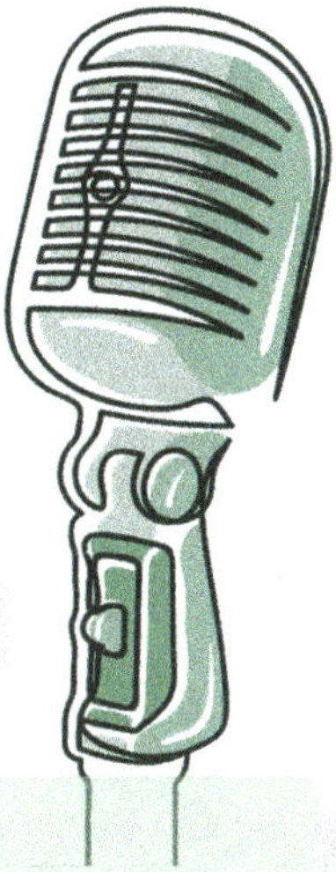

What keeps me grounded?

Micro Self-Care Do More Lists:

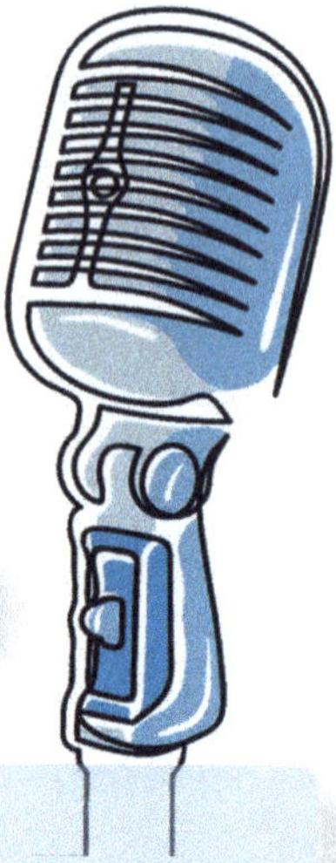

When am I at my best?

Micro Self-Care Do More Lists:

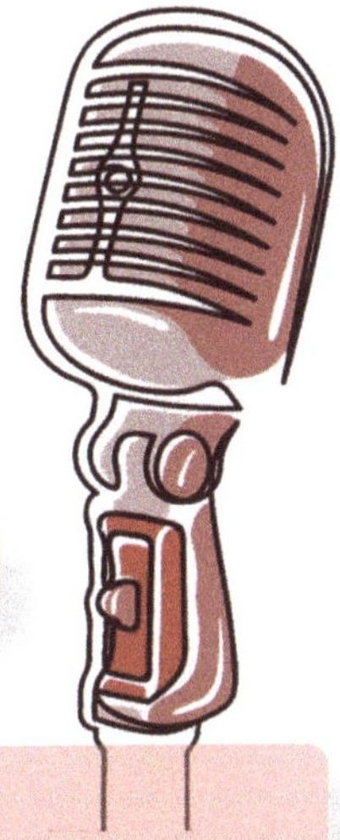

Where do I feel my safest?

"To love oneself is the beginning of a lifelong romance."

-oscar wilde

Change your thoughts and you can change the world.

What does your new thought plan look like; write down goals for each area."

Personal Development

Self Care

Mental Care

day 4

Self-Kindness

Appreciation refers to the act of recognizing and valuing the worth or importance of something or someone. It can be shown in various ways such as expressing gratitude, admiration, or respect towards someone or for something. Appreciation can also refer to an increase in the value of an asset over time, such as a stock or a piece of real estate. (p.329)

Write down 5 things

That you like about yourself!

Ways to Express Self-Kindness

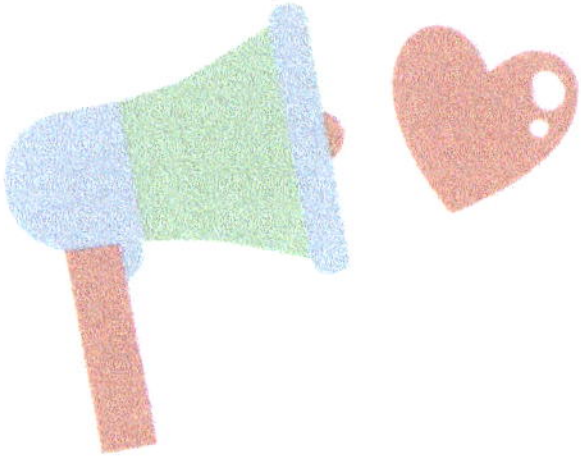

Give yourself a compliment

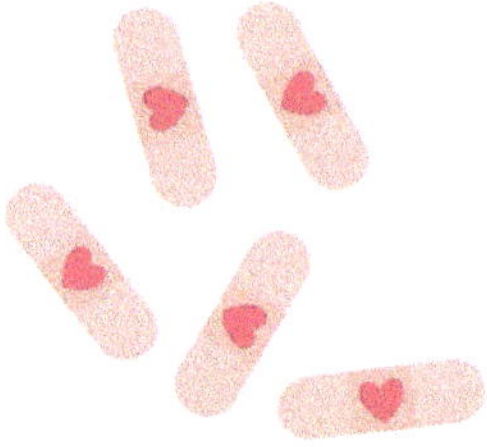

Allow yourself to rest

Make a list of things you are grateful for

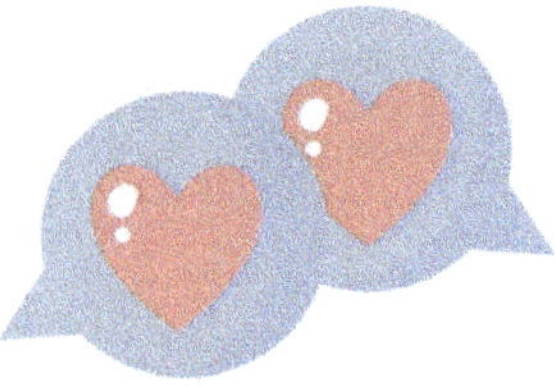

Talk to yourself as you would a friend

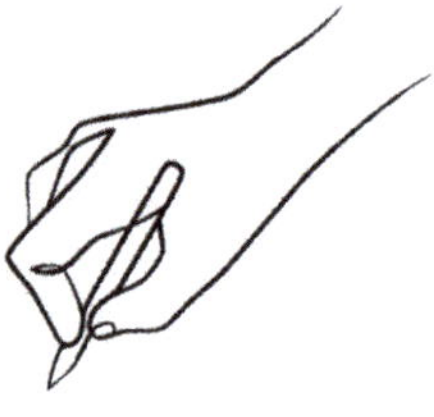

Write down five positive affirmations

Celebrate your small wins

Self-kindness is the act of extending compassion to oneself when one feels inadequate, fails, or suffers in general.

By being kind and accepting of ourselves despite our perceived flaws or mistakes, we can boost our mood and improve our mental health.

Practicing self kindness over time can also create positive patterns and lead to increased resilience.

How can you express self-kindness today?

Appreciation

Ask yourself and write your answers below

WHO do I appreciate right now?

Appreciation

Ask yourself and write your answers below

WHERE can I be appreciated?

Appreciation

Ask yourself and write your answers below

WHAT do I appreciate right now?

Appreciation

Ask yourself and write your answers below

HOW can I cultivate more appreciation in my life?

day 5

Conquering Emotional Adversity

Emotional Adversity is the ability to overcome rigidity, fear, stuck points, and pain by moving into emotionally intelligent behavior. By learning to manage our emotions through regulation and skill development, we can open our minds to growth promoting change and cultivating a present, calm, mindset. (p.332)

How do you take care of your mind, body and soul?

Write specific action words down below:

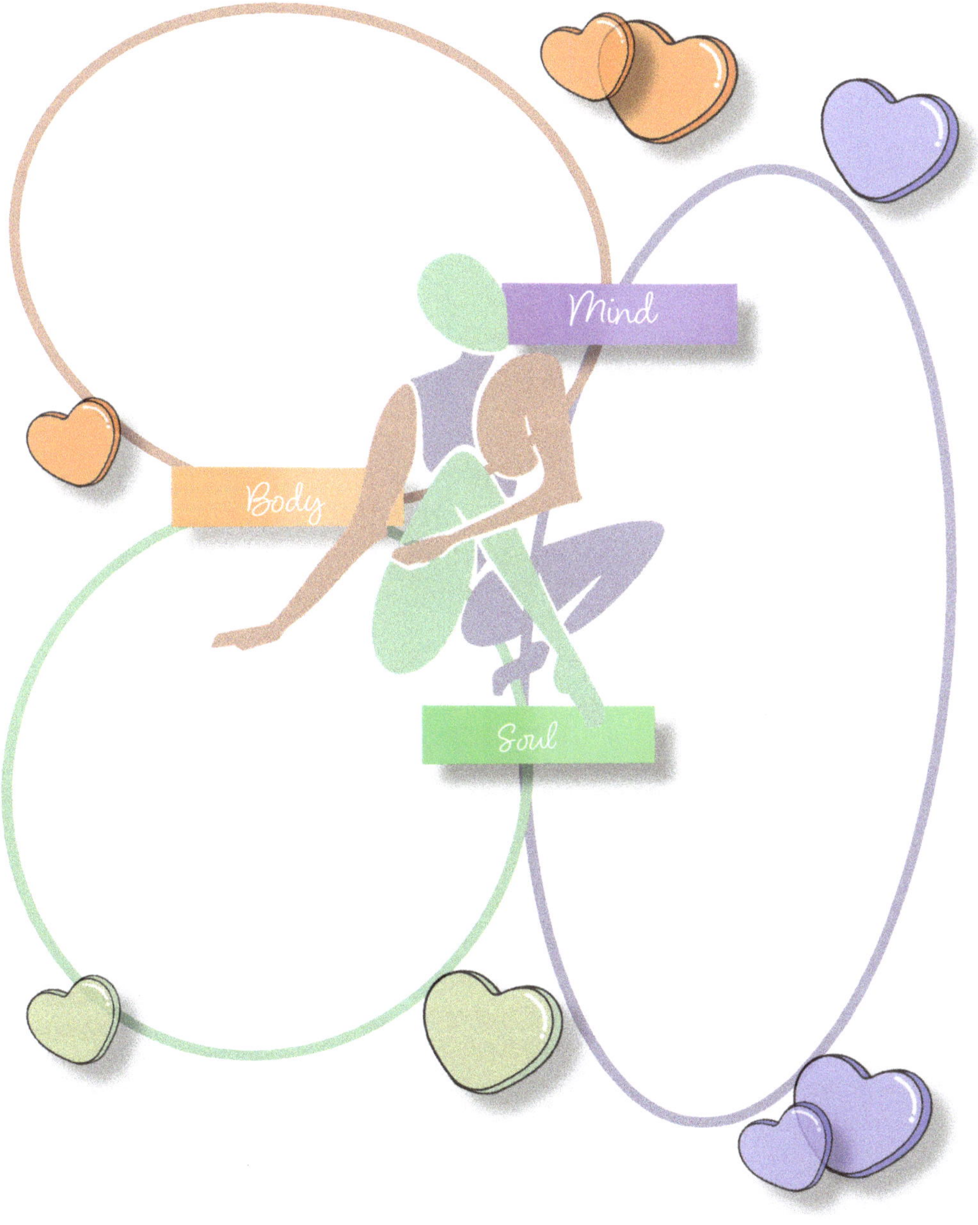

If Today Is Tough...

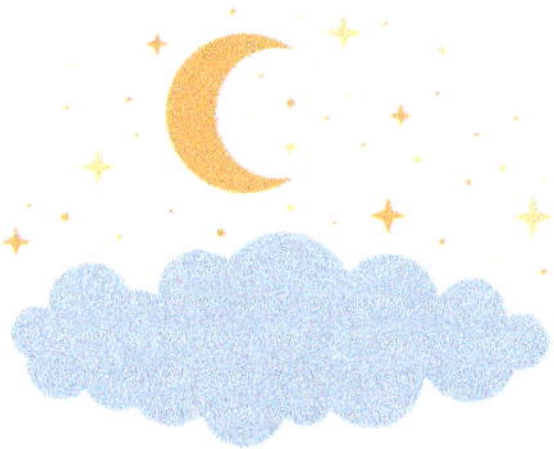

Go for a long drive
and watch the sun set

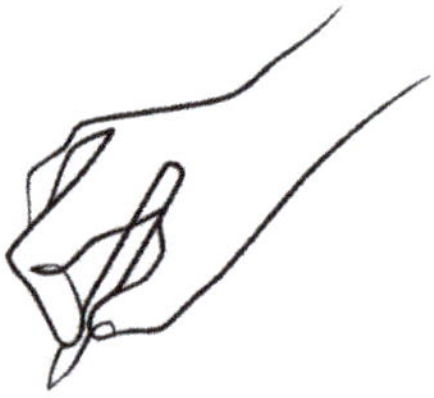

Journal about
something that makes
you grateful

Spend the day
offline and away
from screens

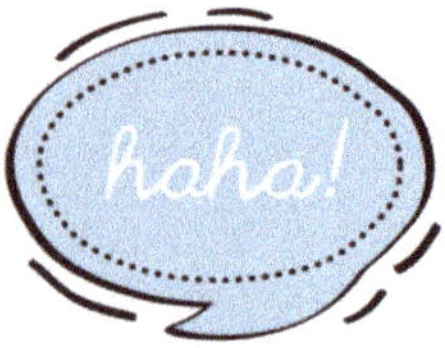

Watch a funny
video or comfort movie

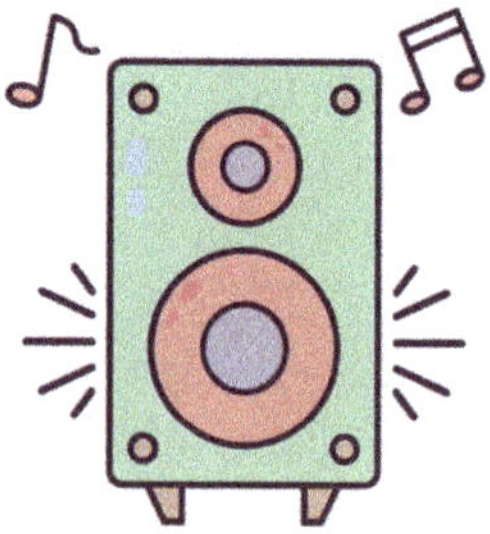

Put on your favorite music
and go for a walk outside

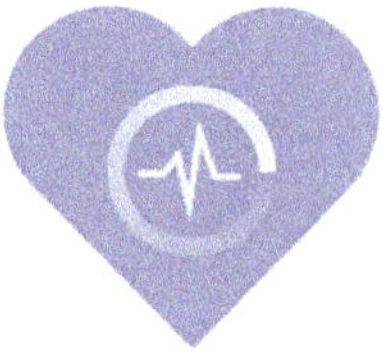

Do a short
mindfulness or
breathing exercise

Here are some self-care activities to do when you are having a tough day!

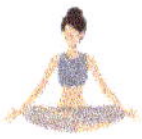

Put away or reduce all distractions if you're feeling overwhelmed or overstimulated!

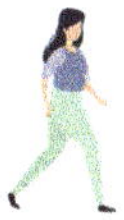

Go on a nature walk to boost your mood and reduce stress.

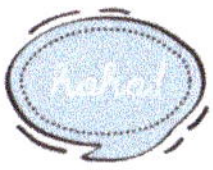

If you need a good laugh, watch a funny show, movie, or video.

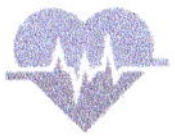

To lower the heart rate and calm the body, try going for a long drive or practicing relaxation techniques.

What can you do today to take care of yourself?

Do you get stuck in negative thinking patterns or have unwanted intrusive thoughts? If so, how...

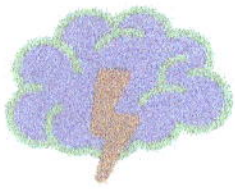

Often when we take our thoughts at face value we get stuck in a cycle of anxiety that feels inescapable.

When you recognize an intrusive thought, try an activity from page 4~ this will help you to reset.

When you do this, it can help you to realize that you are being overly critical of yourself and help you to create a more realistic thought.

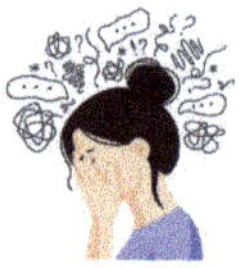

You can also learn to recognize when your thoughts are very unlikely to happen or the worst case scenario, and therefore not worth stressing over.

What do negative or intrusive thoughts look like for you? Spend a few minutes writing down your answers below.

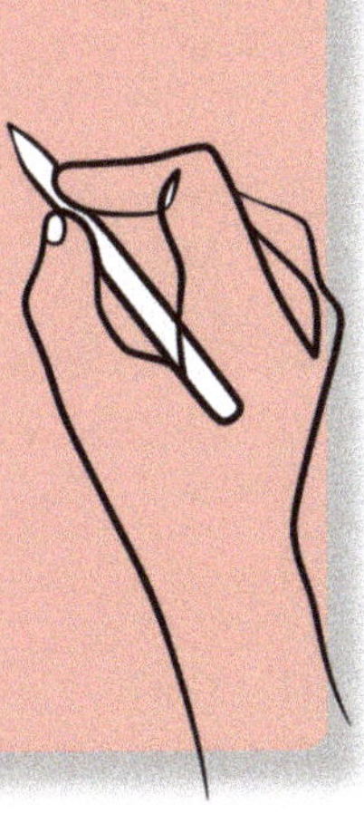

How do you notice these thoughts impact your happiness and self- love?

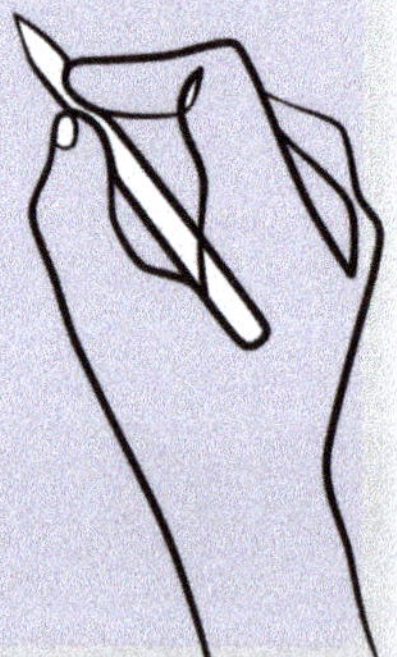

Ways That You Can Begin To Heal

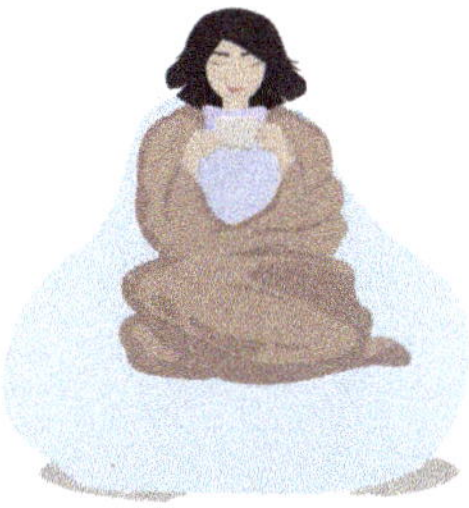

Keeping your environment comfortable

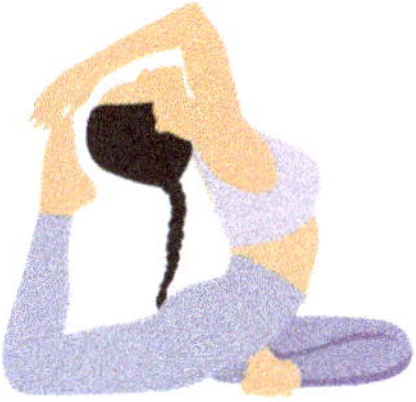

Exercising, walking and getting some fresh air

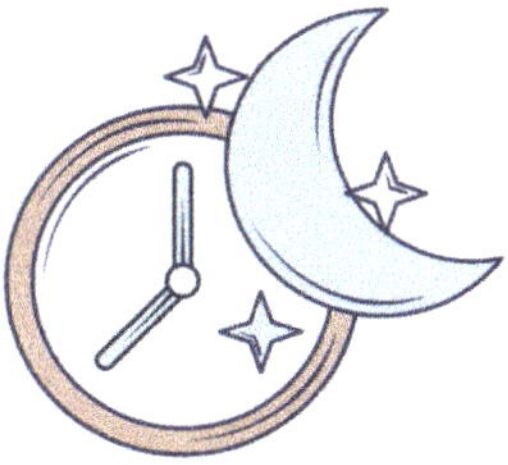

Resting and getting a good night's sleep

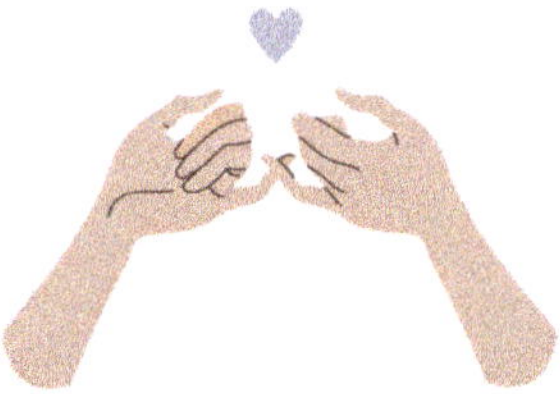

Developing trusting relationships

Drinking something hot or cold to help reset

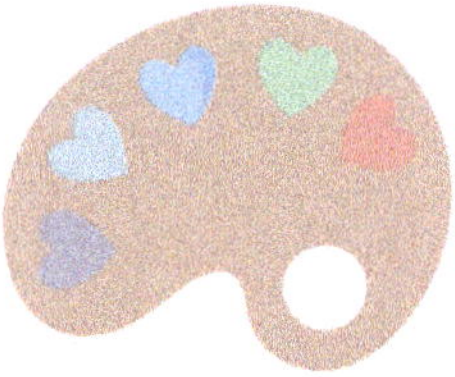

Finding positive outlets

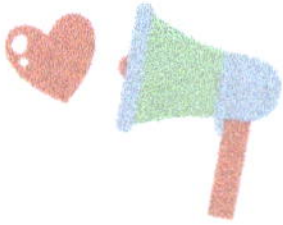

Our emotions can teach us meaningful things about ourselves!

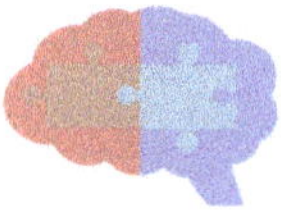

When strong emotions arise try feeling them rather than fighting them.

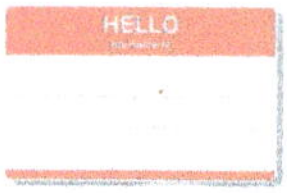

Start by gently naming the emotion you are feeling without judgment.

After this, ask yourself what you may need, and come up with a 3 minute action plan of what you are going to do. Write it here:

Remember that it's okay to experience painful emotions. We all experience them from time to time; treat yourself with kindness.

How will you hold your self accountable to create more kindness towards yourself this week?

day 6

Positive Thinking

Positive Self-talk is speaking to ourselves in a way that is uplifting and kind. Positive self-talk involves offering validation and compassion to ourselves. Although we may experience difficult times, positive self-talk is a great way to avoid getting stuck in negative thought patterns and to instead invest in our well-being by cultivating self-love.

(p.335)

How will you cultivate positive thinking this week?

Setting small goals makes this achievable and cultivates more success!

Daily Affirmations

PRACTICE SAYING THESE ALOUD

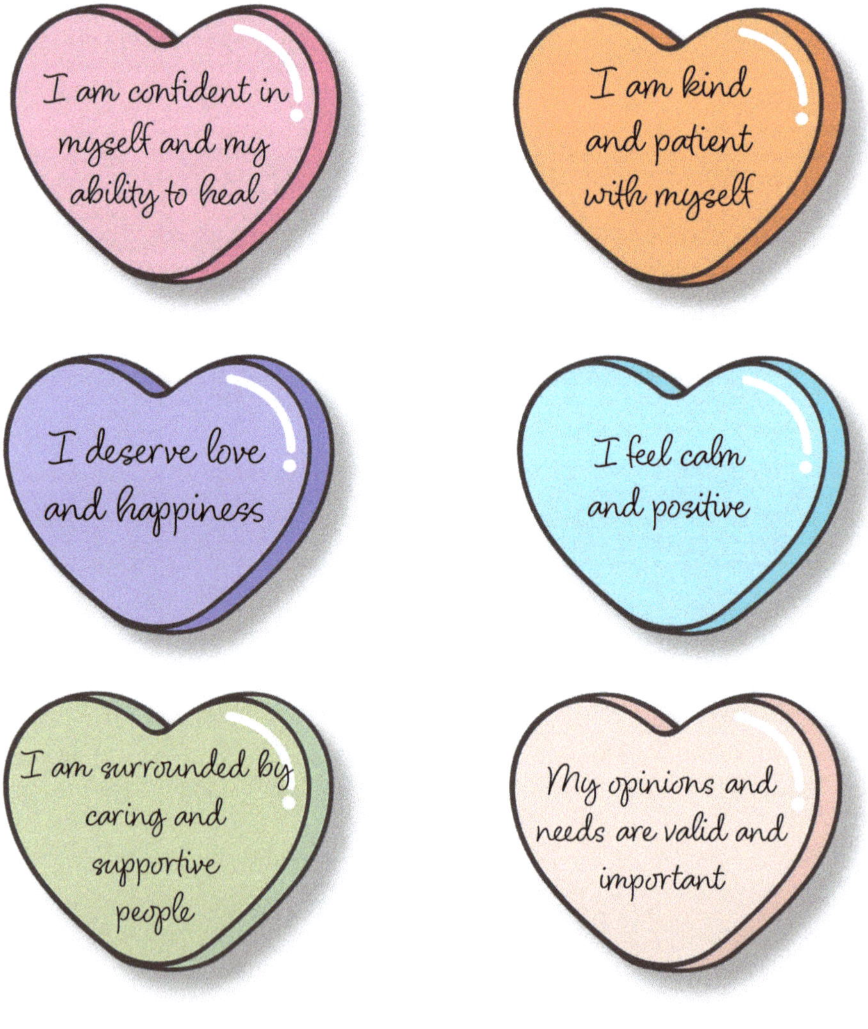

Positive self-talk is an excellent method of practicing self-love and compassion towards oneself.

It helps us to appreciate our positive qualities and build our self-esteem and confidence.

In addition, it can help to effectively counteract our feelings of panic, stress, and doubt.

Try writing down some positive affirmations on sticky notes and put them up on your mirror!

Make a note below of which affirmation is your favorite! Next, write this down below:

Thought Stopping in 6 Steps

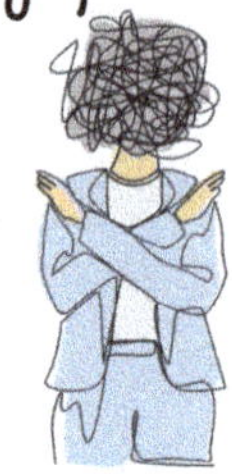

TELL YOURSELF
TO STOP

↓

VISUALIZE A
STOP SIGN

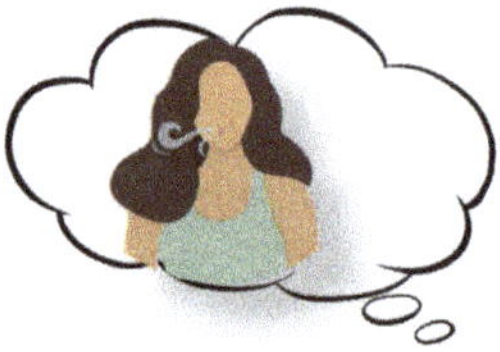

↓

3 BELLY BREATHS
(4X4 BREATHING)

↓

REFRAMING
THOUGHTS

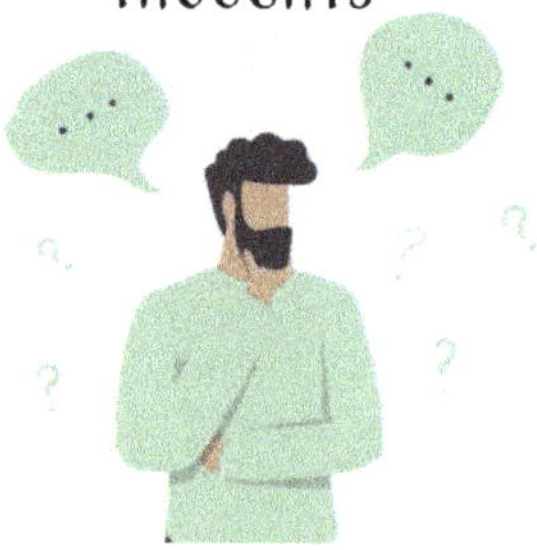

WHAT DO I NEED TO
DO NEXT

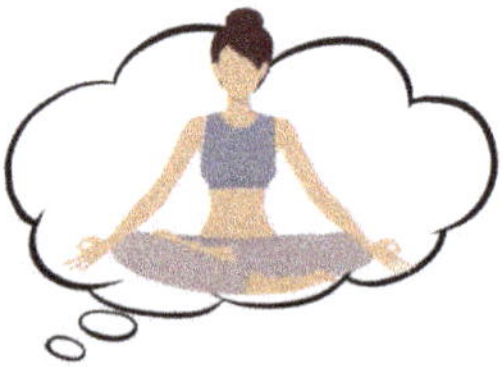

↓

BELLY BREATHS
(4X4 BREATHING)

1. STOP

Move from Flight-Fight-Freeze to Relax-Rest-Digest by imagining a stop sign

2. RESET

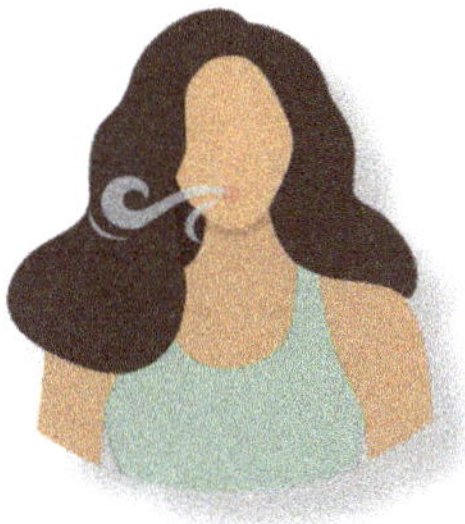

Breathe 3 belly breaths while imagining the reset button

3. CONNECT

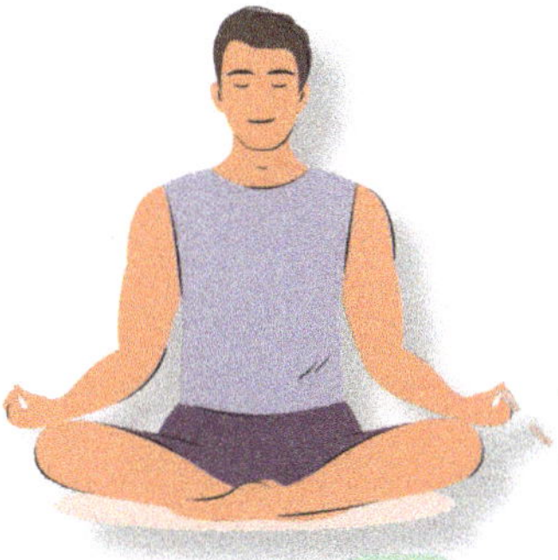

Regain focus and get back into control with thought stopping and becoming present

Reframing Thoughts

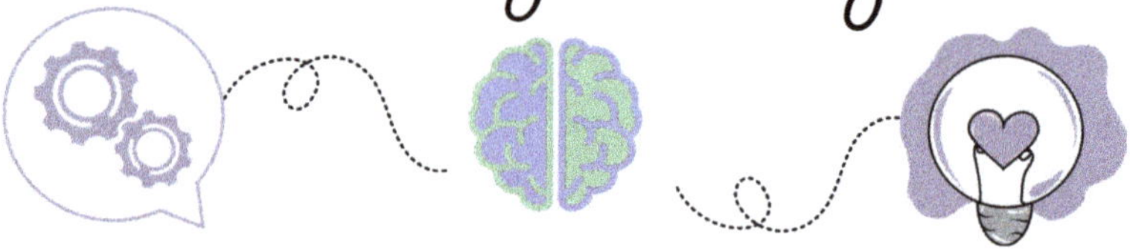

I am (emotion), what I think right now is...

What I feel right now is...

What I believe right now is...

What I want right now is...

What I need right now is...

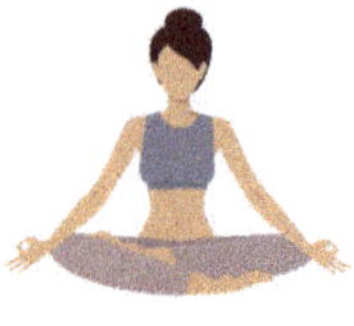

Eg: I am anxious, what I need right now is to take 3 deep breathes and go for a walk. Then I will return the call to my boss.

When I think about changing by thinking, I fear. . .

day 7

Strengthening Coping Skills

Coping is the ability to develop strategies that help us to manage stressful or potentially harmful situations. Healthy coping strategies, such as going for a walk, tapping, listening to music, and lowering stress can help us to reduce the impact of stressful situations by making them more manageable. (p.331)

Challenging a Thought

Might Sound Like...

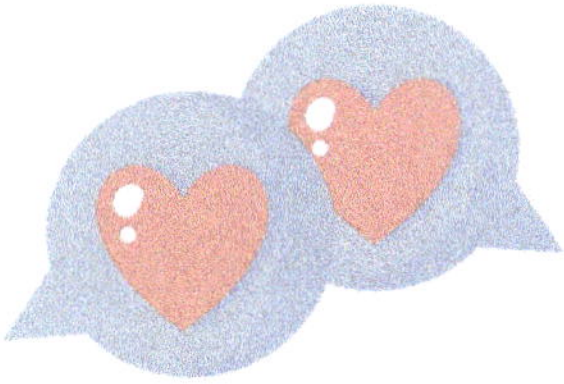

What would I tell a friend who had this thought?

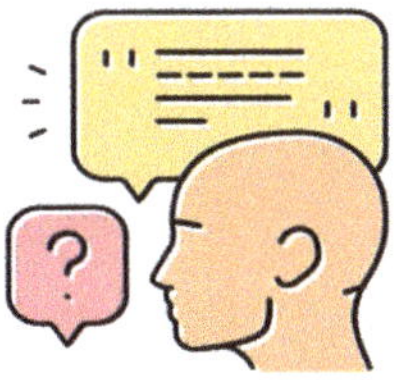

Has this ever happened to me before?

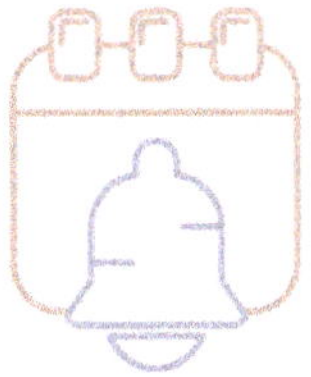

Am I 100% sure that this will happen?

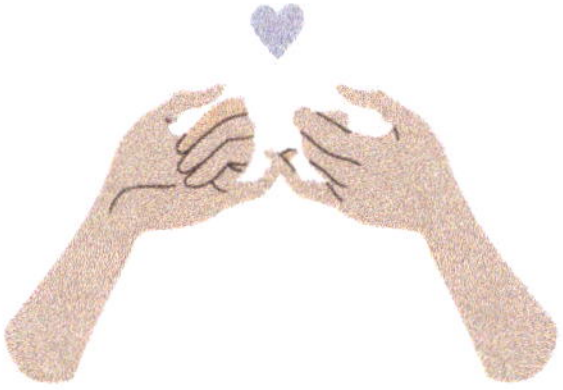

What would a friend say to this thought?

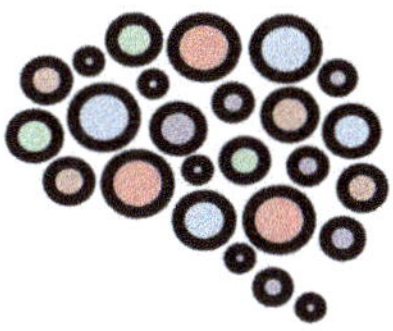

Am I catastrophizing?

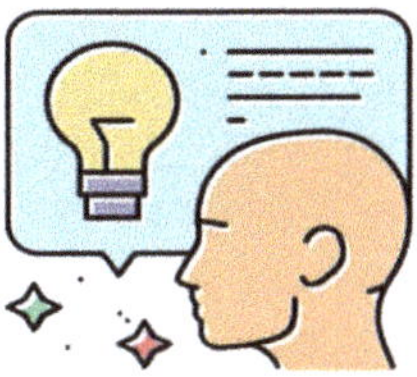

Is this a fact or is it a false belief?

Which thought comes up repeatedly throughout most days for you? Write it down below, then answer the questions on the following pages.

What are the facts? How often has this ever happened to me before? What are the facts versus fiction with this thought?

What would a friend say to this thought?

Am I 100% sure that this will happen?
Prove it to yourself below:

Coping Thoughts

Might Sound Like...

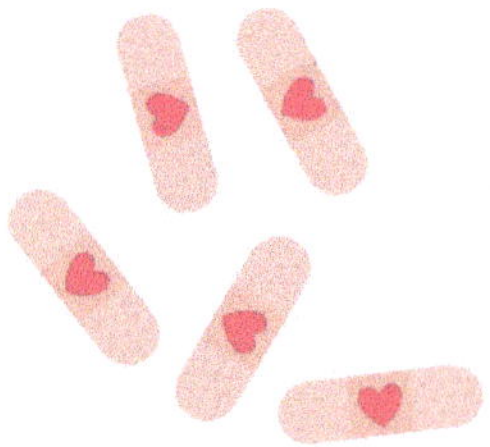

I am worthy of healing and recovery.

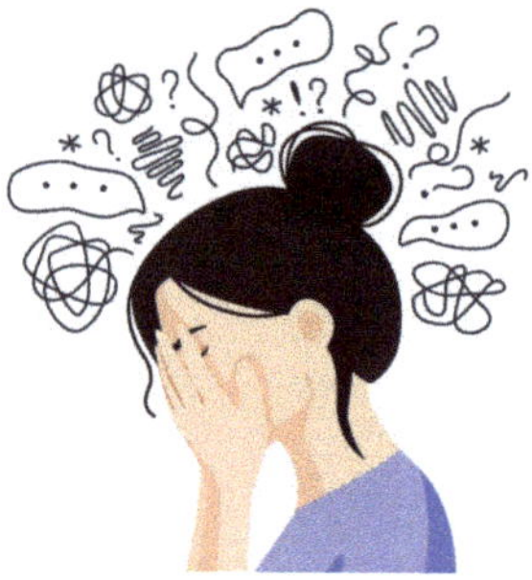

These feelings are uncomfortable but they will pass.

This hurts, so I need to be extra kind to myself.

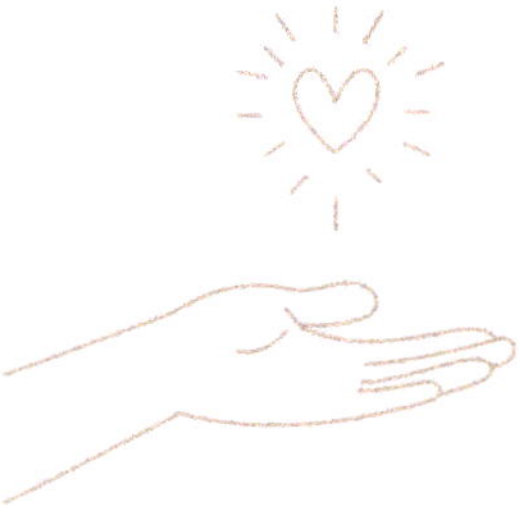

I've dealt with harder situation sand I know things will get better.

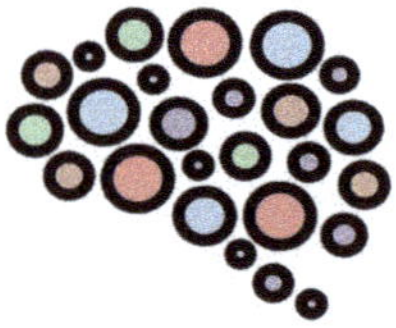

Just because I'm thinking something doesn't mean it's true.

Not everything will go my way, but I can control how I respond.

Make a list of your coping thoughts

Reframe your negative statements into positive statements. Write down one sentence that you can recall, repeat, and create actionable thinking based on your NEW coping strategy.

day 8

Feelings Are Not Facts

Feelings are subjective experiences that arise from our emotions, thoughts, and physical sensations. They can be positive or negative, ranging from subtle to overwhelming. Common feelings include happiness, sadness, anger, fear, joy, love, and contentment. Feelings can influence our behavior, decisions, and overall well-being. (p.333)

Feelings Are Not Facts

Embrace all of your thoughts: the good, the bad, the ugly, the lovely! These are your feelings, not facts. These thoughts do not define you. They are just thoughts! Lean into them, recognize them, allow them to wash over you; then, let them go!

YOU can control how you respond to your feelings, they do not control YOU!

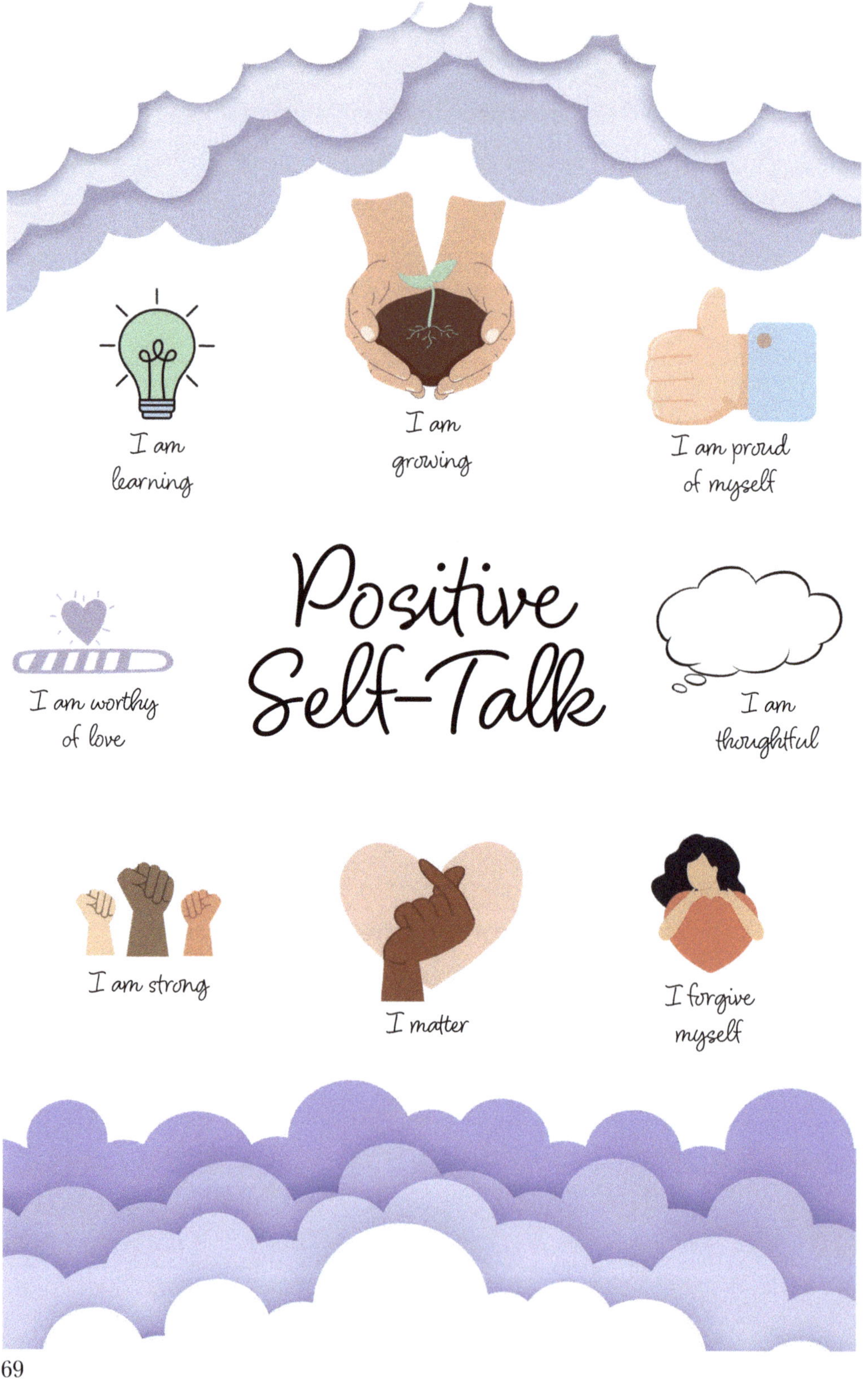
I am learning
I am growing
I am proud of myself
Positive Self-Talk
I am worthy of love
I am thoughtful
I am strong
I matter
I forgive myself

Positively reframing negative thoughts is one helpful way to cope with intrusive thoughts, poor self-esteem, depression, and anxiety.

When rational self-talk is practiced and learned, your brain takes over and it automatically occurs.

You can actually change your brain chemistry by incorporating more positive thoughts and affirmations into your daily routine.

Through this practice you will be more likely to think kind thoughts automatically in the future. This will encourage a positive pattern in your life of self-kindness and self-compassion.

Try speaking to yourself in a kind way today! What would you say?

What's your reframing mantra today?

Reframing our negative beliefs

with empowering "I" STATEMENTS

I get to

Reframing our negative beliefs

with empowering "I" STATEMENTS

I can take control by

Reframing our negative beliefs

with empowering "I" STATEMENTS

I'm loveable because

Reframing our negative beliefs

with empowering "I" STATEMENTS

I celebrate me by

Reframing our negative beliefs

with empowering "I" STATEMENTS

I choose to take a new path by doing

Reframing our negative beliefs

with empowering "I" STATEMENTS

I will make this shift now by

Reframing our negative beliefs

with empowering "I" STATEMENTS

I am amazing when I

Reframing our negative beliefs

with empowering "I" STATEMENTS

I love me when I'm

Reframing our negative beliefs

with empowering "I" STATEMENTS

I'm proud of

Reframing our negative beliefs

with empowering “I” STATEMENTS

I will stand up for myself by

Reframing our negative beliefs

with empowering "I" STATEMENTS

I can always count on myself to

Reframing our negative beliefs

with empowering "I" STATEMENTS

When I say NO to

I show myself love!

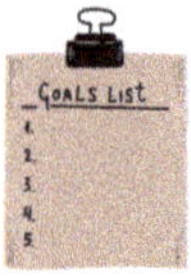

It's important that we pay attention to our negative thoughts and try challenging them with more positive or realistic thoughts instead.

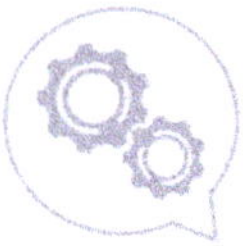

Creating new thinking habits can help us change our brain chemistry and lead to more automatically occurring positive thoughts in the future.

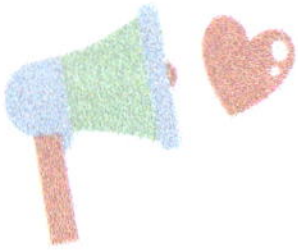

Remember to speak kindly to yourself and to be gentle, especially when you are experiencing painful emotions or going through a tough time.

Be your own biggest supporter! Just because something goes wrong, it does not mean you're a failure. Attempt to recognize things you are good at or times where you did something really awesome.

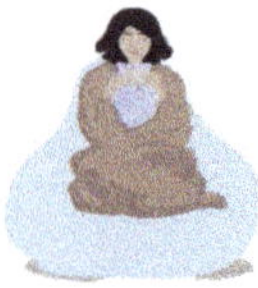

Lastly, don't get down on yourself. Everyone has bad days, don't be too critical of yourself. Accept your feelings and allow yourself to rest without being too judgmental about the way you're feeling.

Feeling are not Facts

YOU can control how you respond to your feelings, they do not control YOU!

YOU can control your response by naming your feelings and reframing your truth!

I feel...	My truth...

day 9

All Bodies Are Bikini Bodies

Body positivity is a philosophy that promotes the acceptance and celebration of all bodies, regardless of their size, shape,or appearance; encouraging individuals to embrace their bodies as they are. Body positivity involves promoting self-love, self-care, and self-acceptance, and rejecting the idea that there is one "ideal" body type or shape. (p.330)

SOMETIMES IF IT'S NOT HARD, CHALLENGING, AND MAYBE EVEN PAINFUL, THEN IT'S NOT GROWING!

Body Acceptance

Might Sound Like...

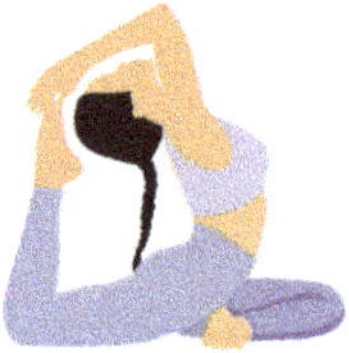

Exercising in a way that makes you personally happy.

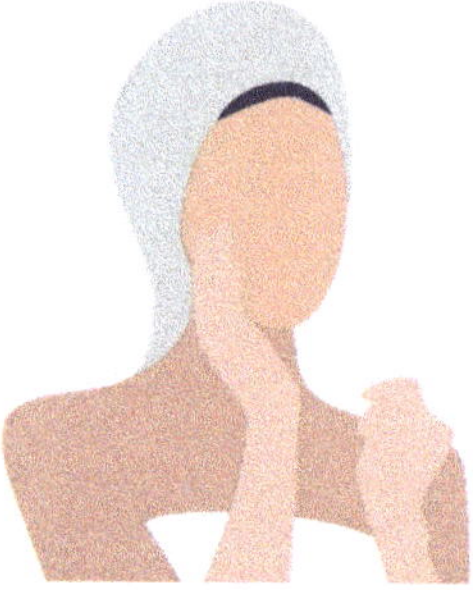

Doing something nice for your body.

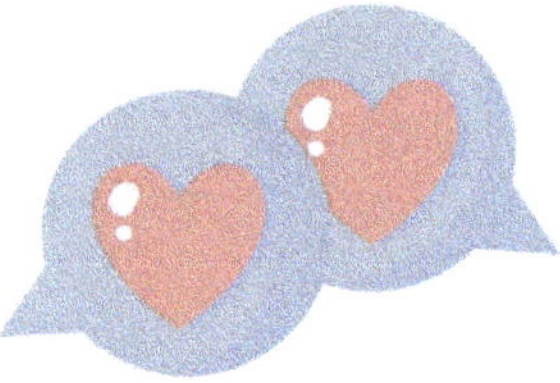

Thinking of five great things that your body helps you do.

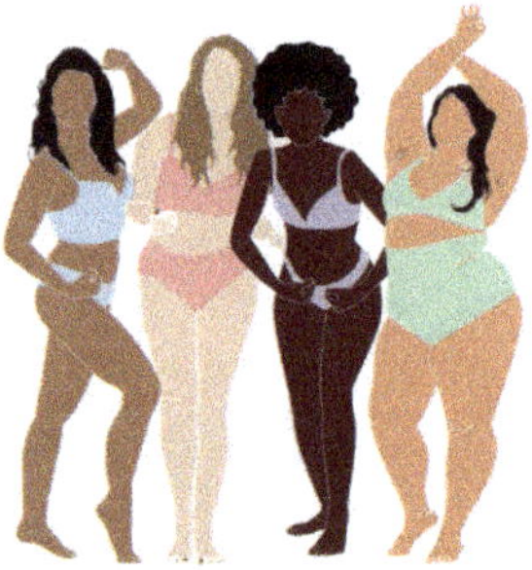

Understanding that a healthy body can look different for everyone.

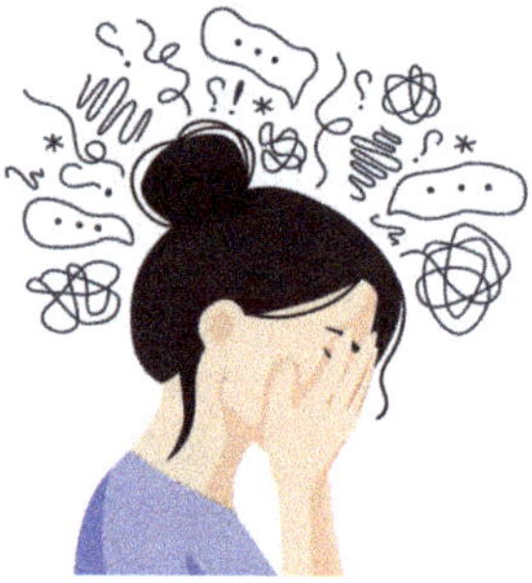

Challenging unhelpful thoughts and reframing them into positive ones.

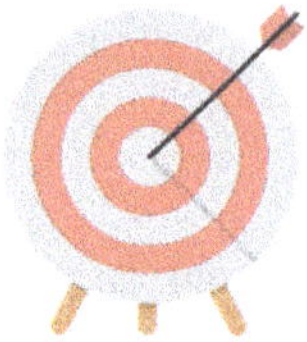

Setting realistic goals for yourself and your body.

It's important to remember that your body is worthy of respect, and that you are worthy of love and happiness regardless of your body size.

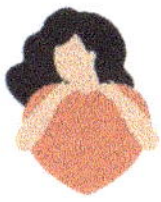

Some ways to counter unrealistic media examples and to promote positive mental health are to practice body acceptance and body positivity.

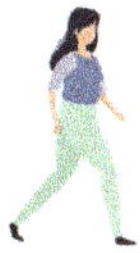

Body positivity is being proud of your body and viewing it and others positively regardless of the societal standards about ideal body shape or size.

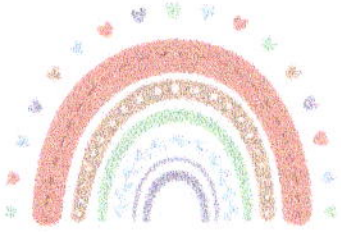

Body acceptance is the process of accepting your body even if you are not completely satisfied with every aspect of it. They are both beneficial in redefining societal standards and our ideas of wellness and health.

Today my body will be worthy because...

Reminder That You Don't Deserve To

Feel Ashamed Of

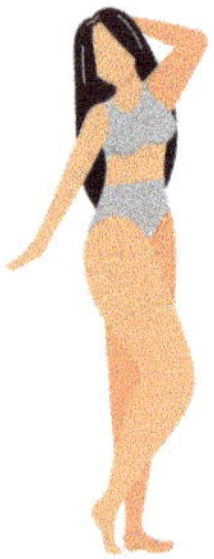

Stretch marks

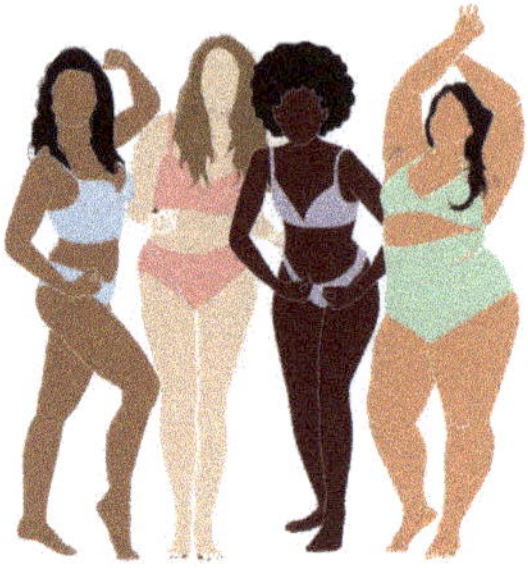

Body shape or size

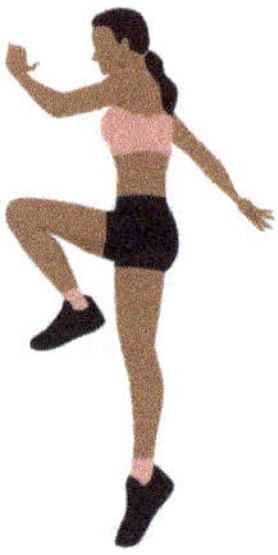

A thigh gap/ or no thigh gap

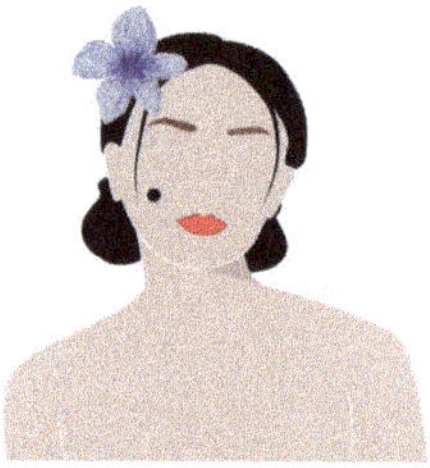

Moles

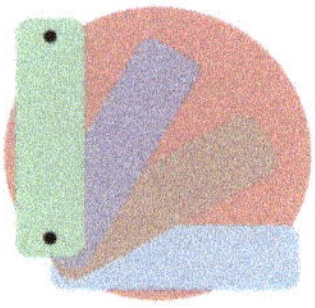

Skin discoloration

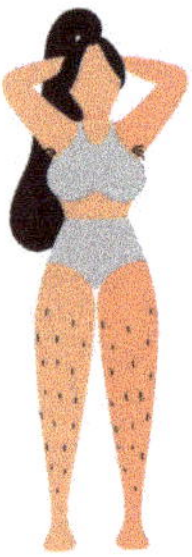

Body hair

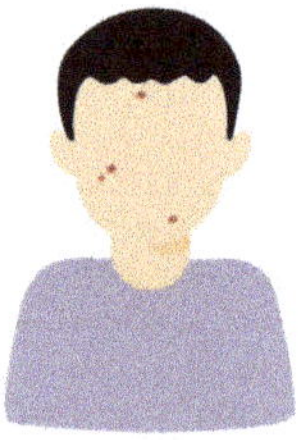

Blemishes

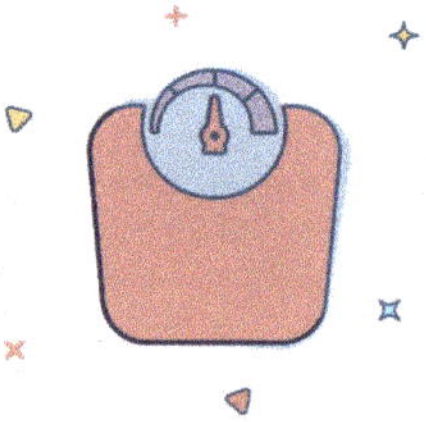

Any fat on your body

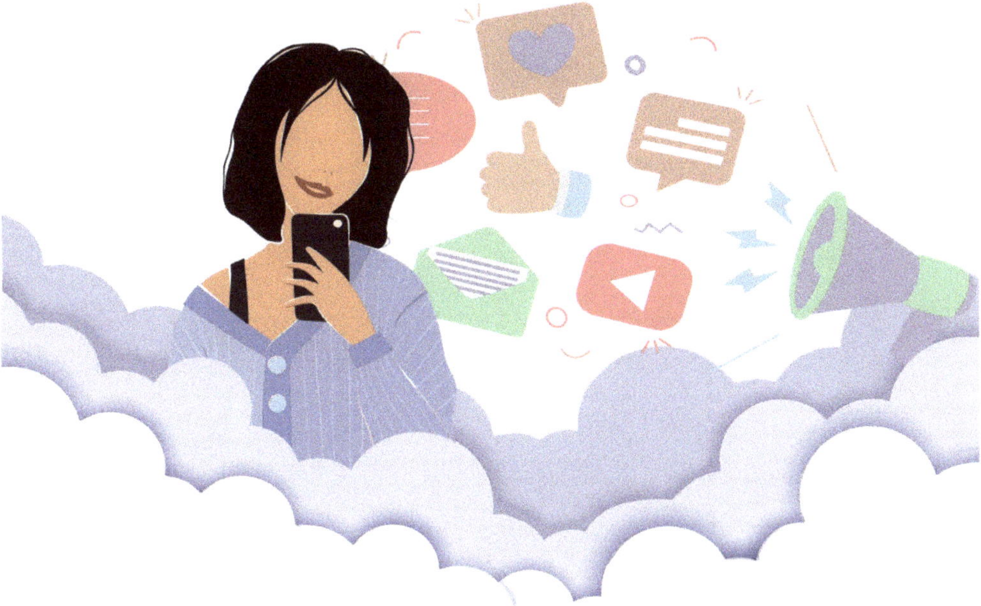

Selfie Challenge

1. TAKE A PICTURE-NO FILTER!

2. POST IT

3. HOW DO YOU FEEL?

> "YOUR BEAUTY IS ALLOWING YOUR INNER SELF TO SHINE BRIGHT LIKE THE STAR YOU ARE!"

Progressive Relaxation

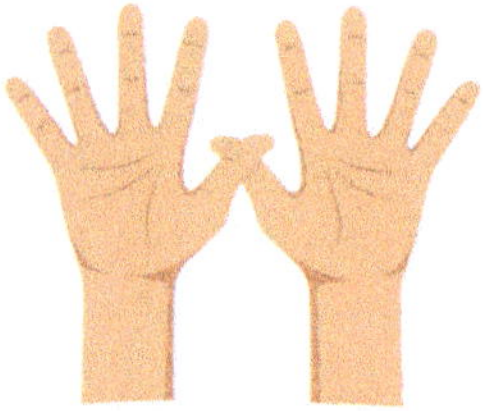

Spread your fingers:
open and close for
slowly for 5 seconds

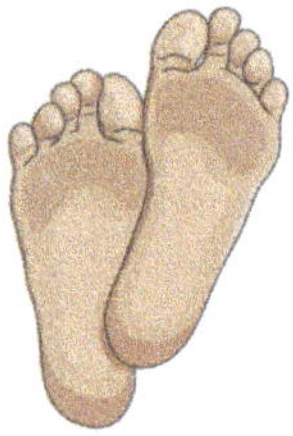

Spread your toes:
open and close for
slowly for 5 seconds

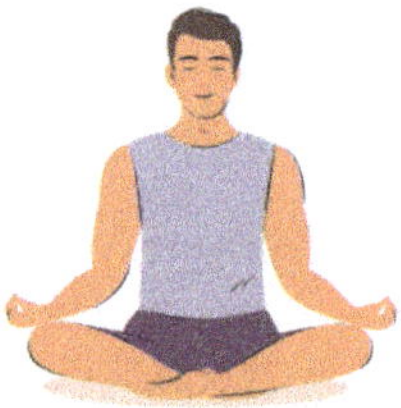

Spread your heart:
5 Big, slow belly
breaths

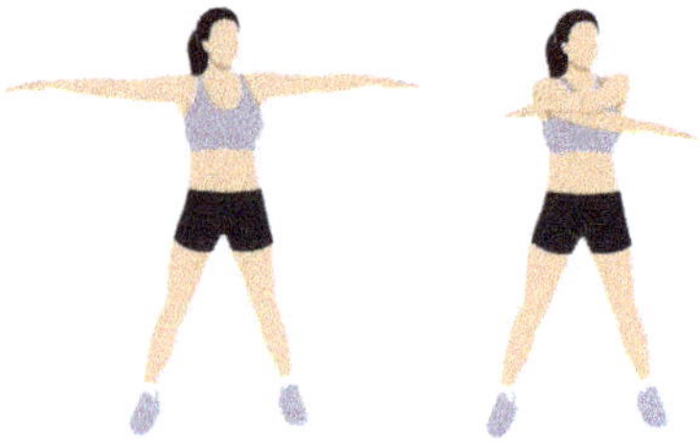

Spread your arms wide:
open and close for
slowly for 5 seconds

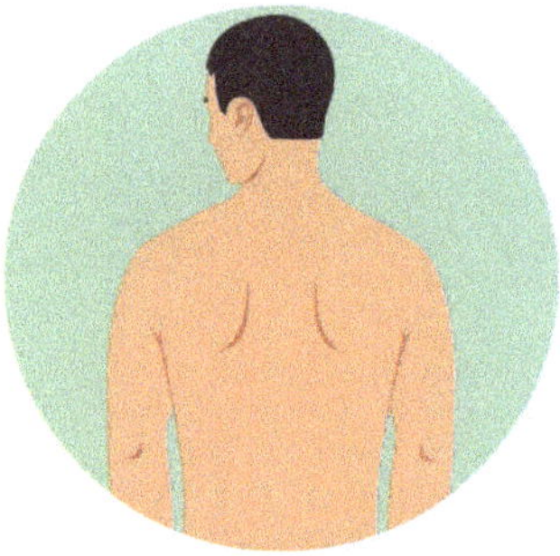

Spread your arms wide
and pull your
shoulders back:
squeeze and release slowly
for 5 seconds

What did you notice in your body when you did this?

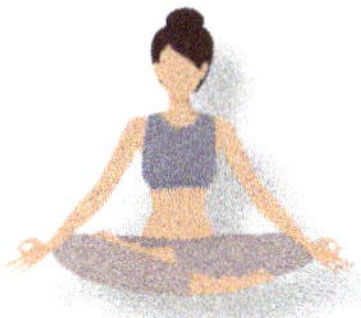

DO YOU FEEL LIGHTER?

On a scale of 0-10, how much lighter do you feel? (0 not at all; 10 feel 100% lighter). Why did you give yourself this rating?

0 —————————————————— 10

day

10

Positive Energy Building

Stress Management consists of strategies that help to manage stress on a day to day basis over time. When we are feeling stressed out, these strategies and coping skills can help us to reduce our stressors by establishing a sense of calm, stimulate relaxation and improve mood. (p.336)

What do I notice about my daily energy levels?

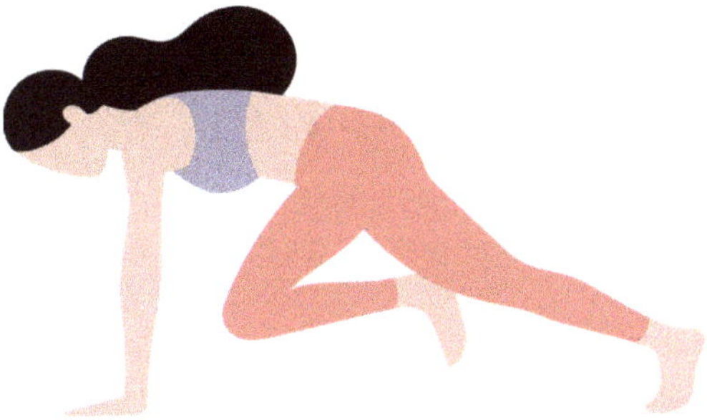

Energy Drainers

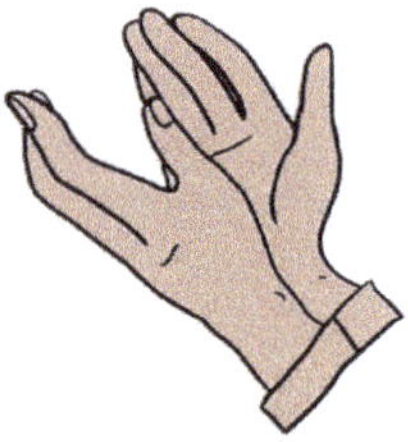

People pleasing

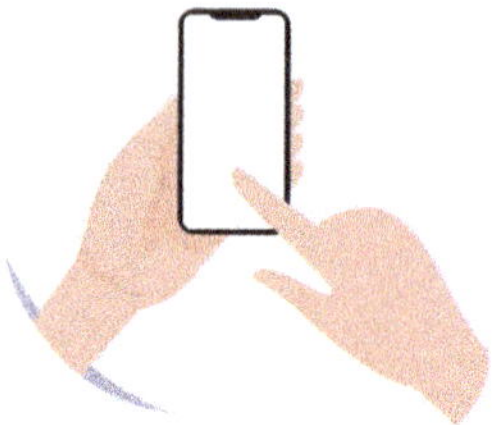

Screen time

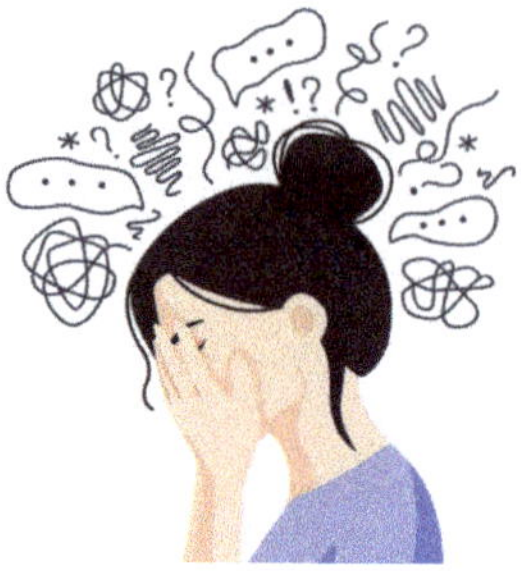

Overthinking

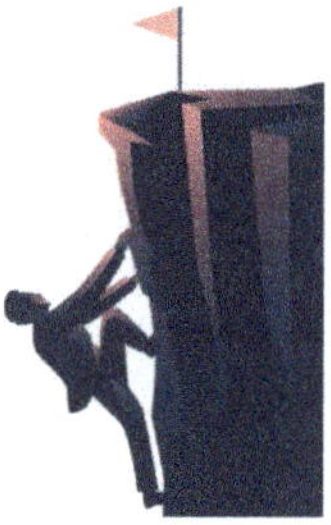

Unrealistic goals

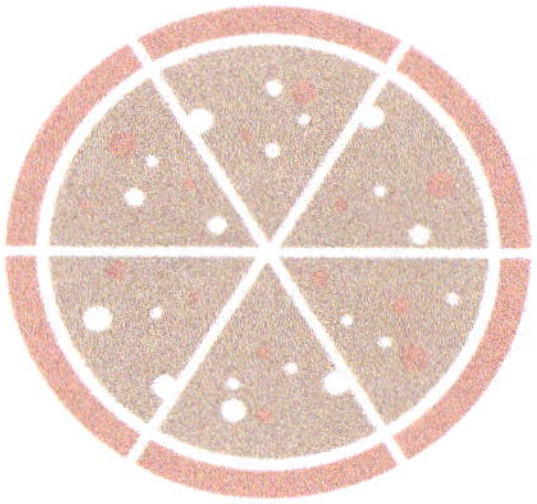

Junk food

Dehydration

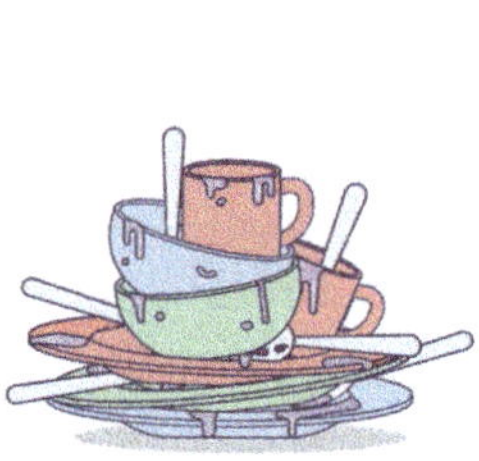

Clutter

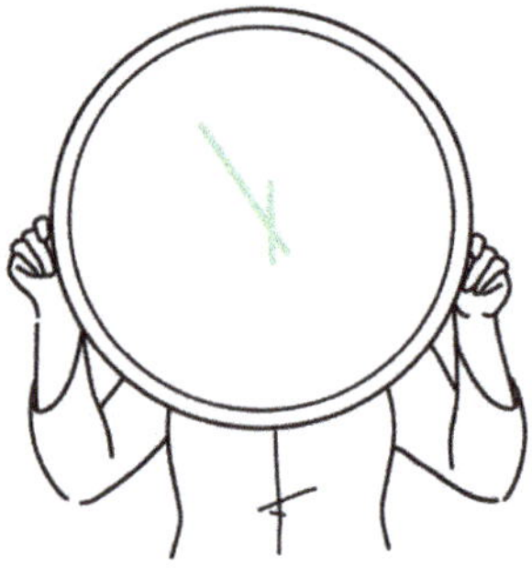

Living in the past

Inactivity

Energy Givers

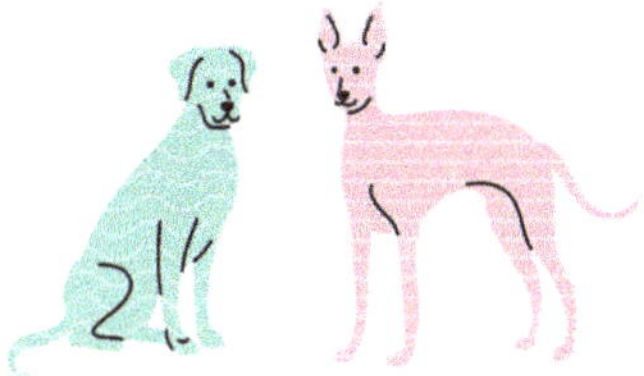

Pets

Sleep

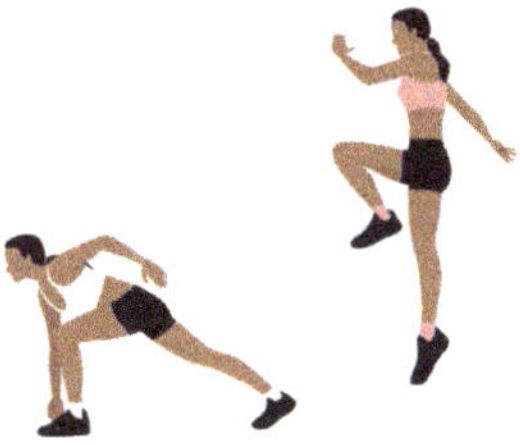

Exercise

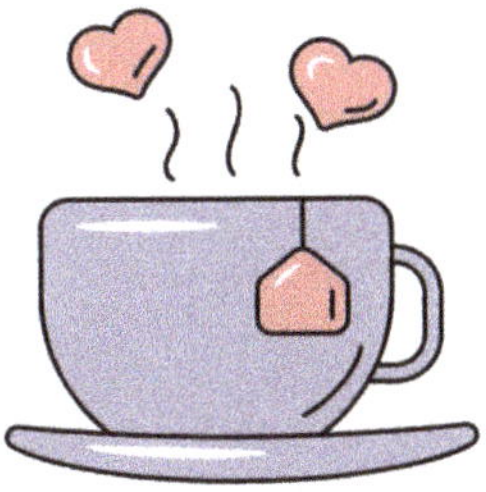

Tea

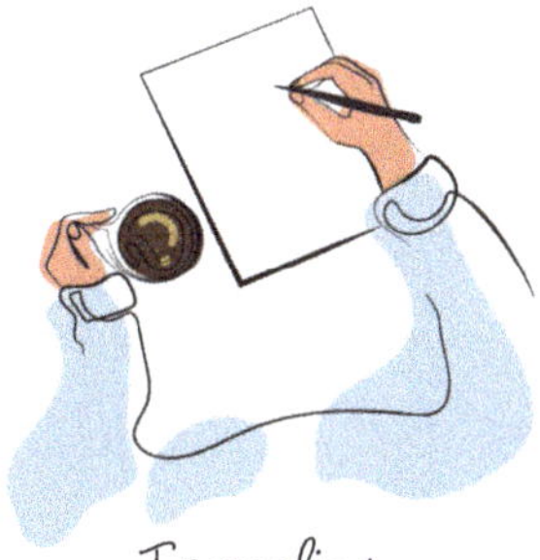

Journaling

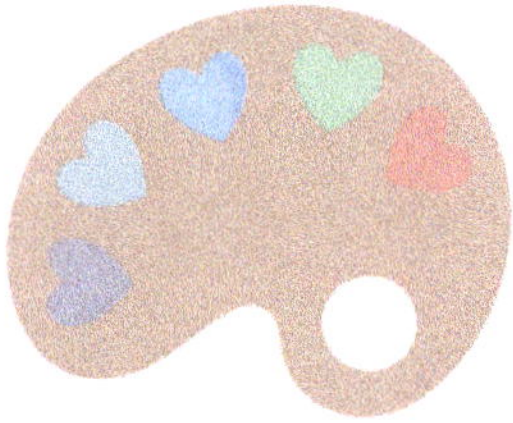

Art/creativity

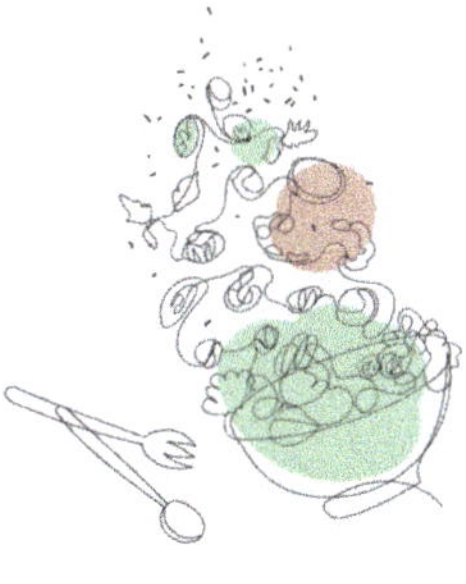

Cooking

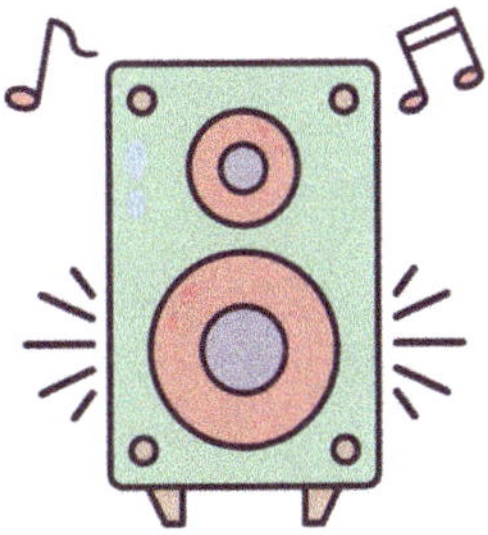

Music

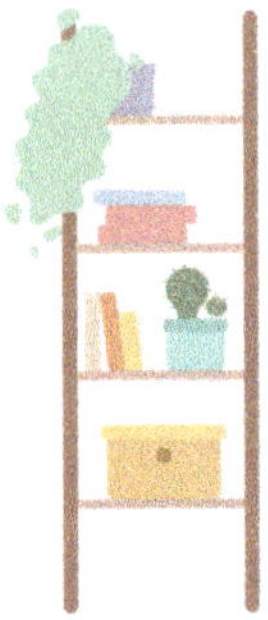

Decluttering

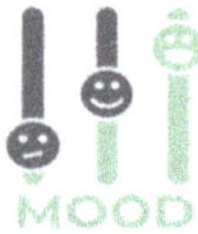

Energy drainers are activities that drain our energy.

It's important to be aware of what activities are draining our energy, because if not dealt with, over time they can accumulate and lead to decreased mood and burnout.

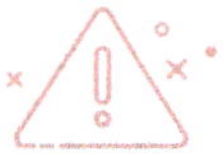

Some common energy drainers are people pleasing, overthinking, and setting unrealistic goals.

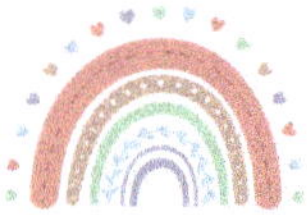

A good balance of energy drainers and givers is crucial. Energy givers such as sunlight, exercise, and meaningful connections can help to mitigate these effects and recharge our battery.

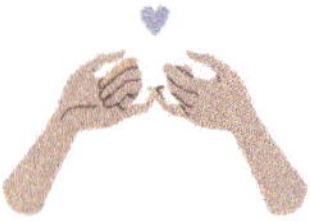

Engaging in energy givers and understanding what drains you will enable you to reclaim this energy and maintain positive mental health.

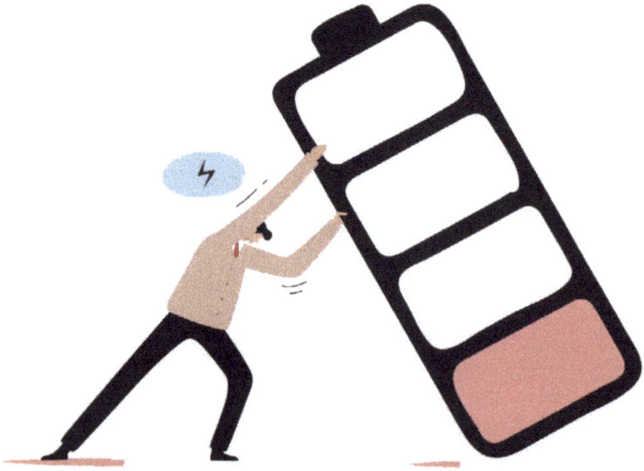

What are the energy drainers that you find zap your energy daily?

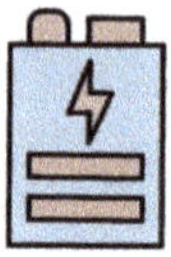

Energy givers are those activities that help you recharge your battery.

Energy givers are a great way to cope with stress, overwhelm, and anxiety.

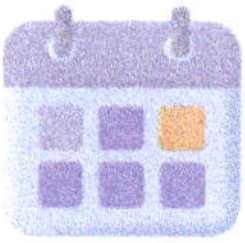

Maintaining a good balance of energy givers and drainers within your schedule is crucial.

By incorporating energy givers into your routine you can help prevent burnout and increase your resilience to stressors.

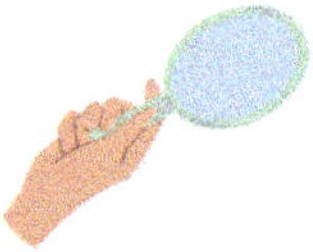

Reflect on what activities you like to engage in when you feel like your social battery is running out or you feel exhausted.

?

What feels most calming and restorative for you?

How can you incorporate these activities into your daily schedule?

What are the energy givers that you find boost your energy daily?

Ways That Stress Shows Up In The Body

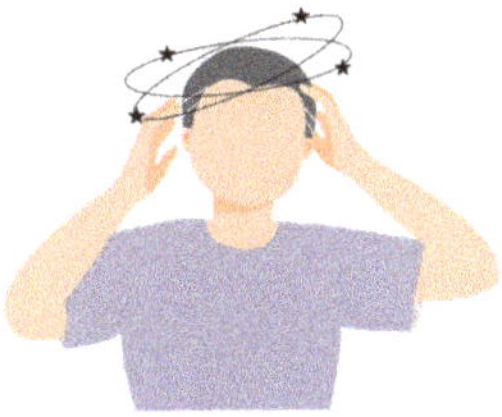

Dizziness

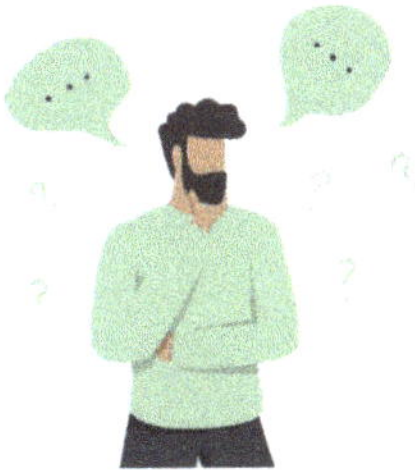

Anxiety

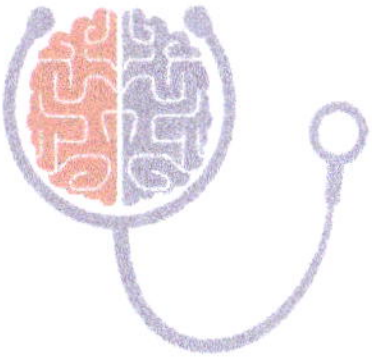

Headaches

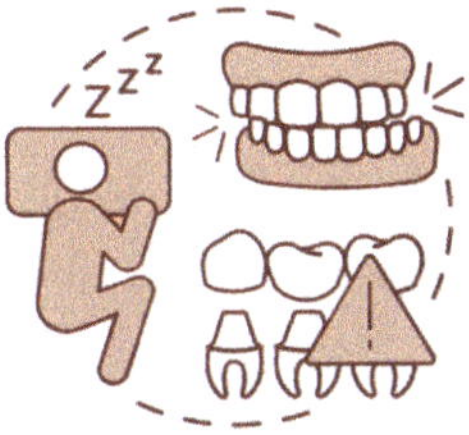

Teeth grinding

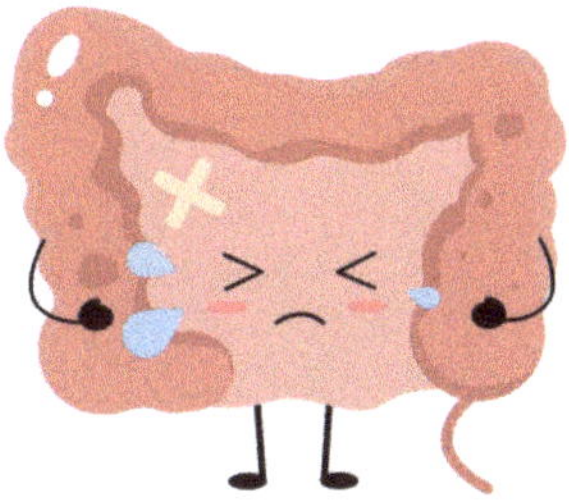

Gut issues

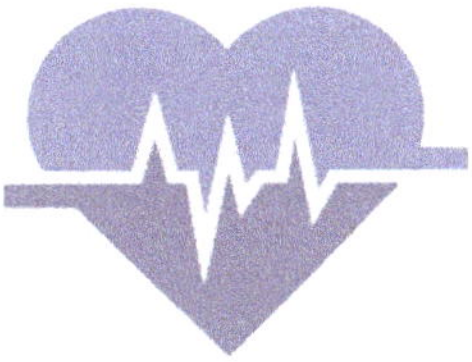

Racing heart

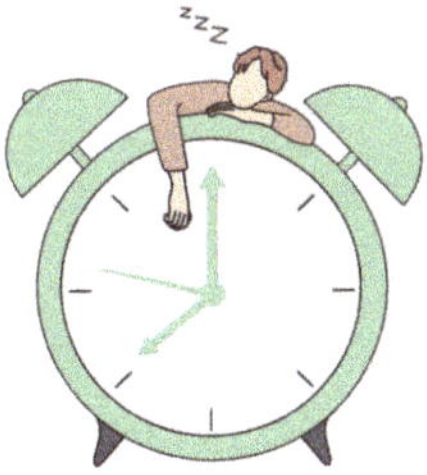

Fatigue / low energy

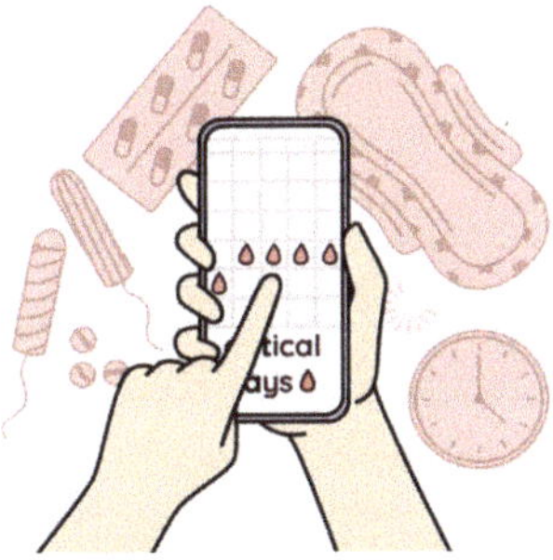

Irregular periods

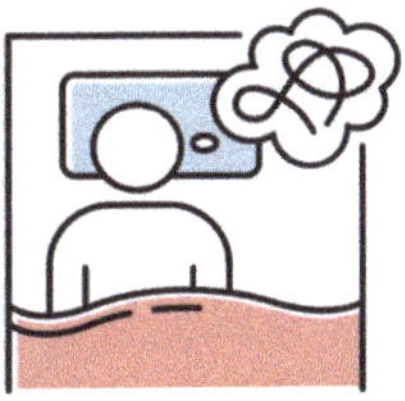

Sleep issues

Creating a good ENERGY practice is one step closer to SELF-LOVE

Energy Givers	Energy Drainers

"Just do what works for you, because there will always be somebody who thinks differently."

–Michelle Obama

day 11

Regaining Control

Boundaries refer to the limits or guidelines that individuals set for themselves in response to others about what is acceptable behavior or treatment when in relationships. Boundaries can be physical, emotional, mental, intimate, professional or spiritual, and can vary depending on the individual and the situation.

(p.331)

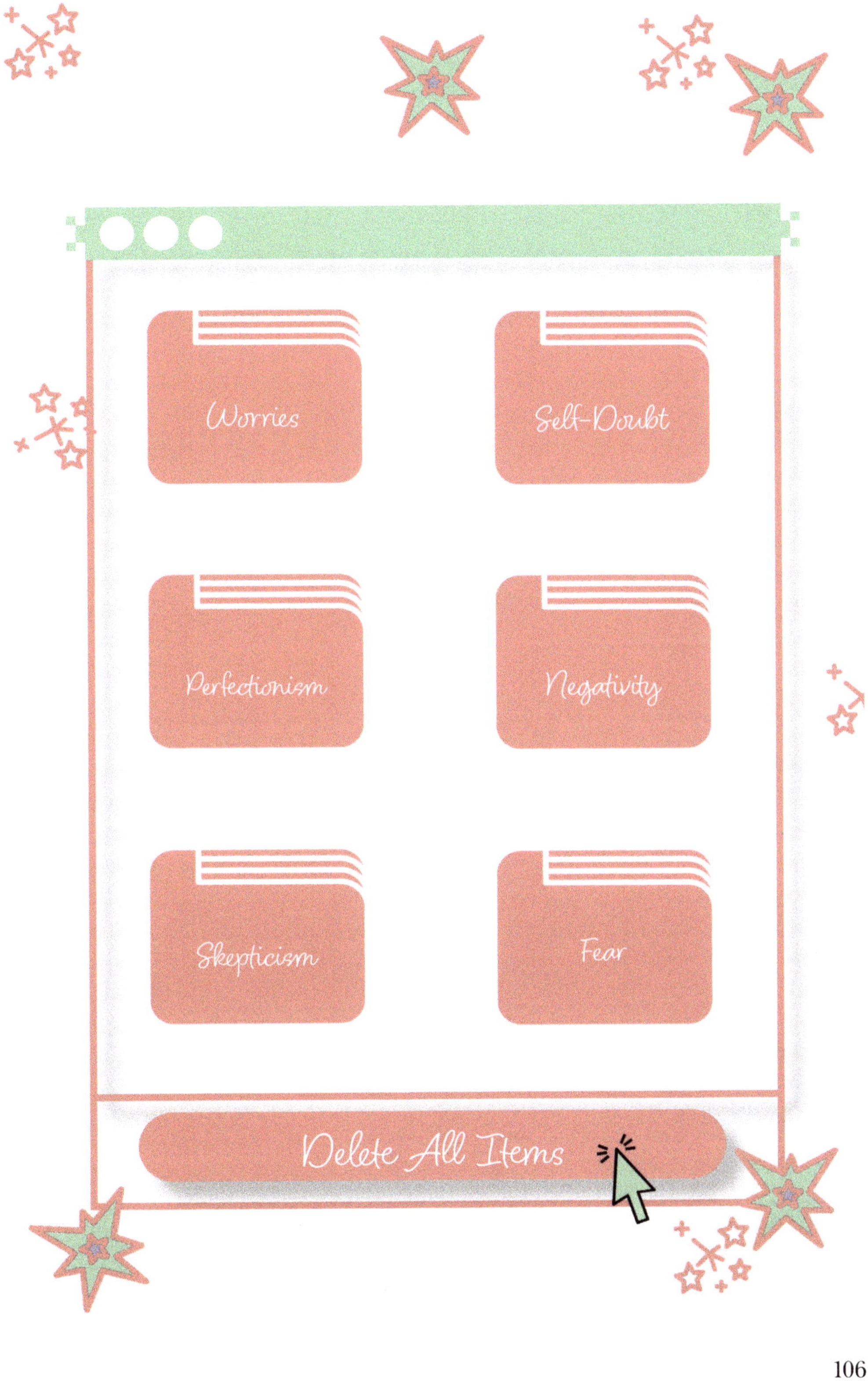
Worries
Self-Doubt
Perfectionism
Negativity
Skepticism
Fear
Delete All Items

Ways to Get Unstuck

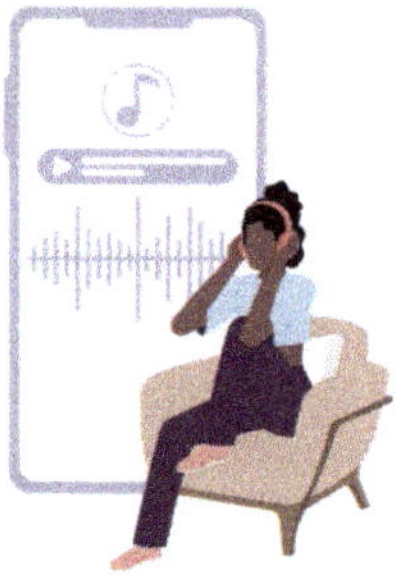

Change your
song playlist

Start working on
a new habit

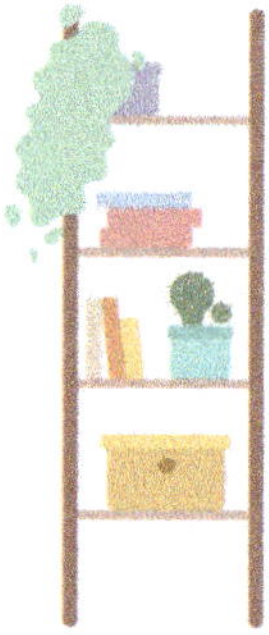

Redecorate your space

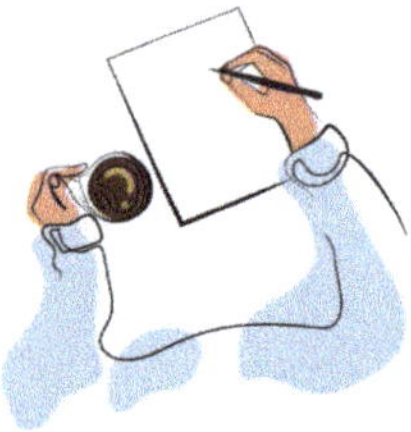

Start journaling daily

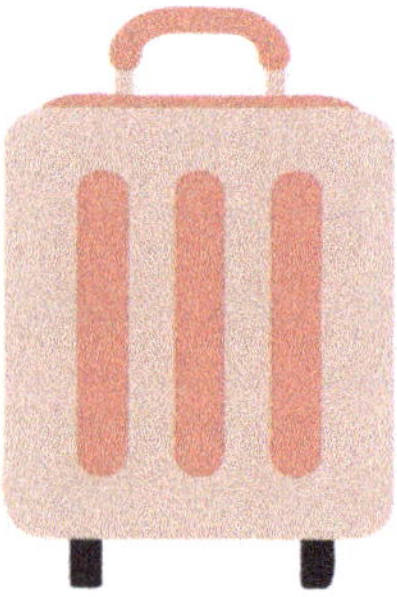

Plan a weekend trip

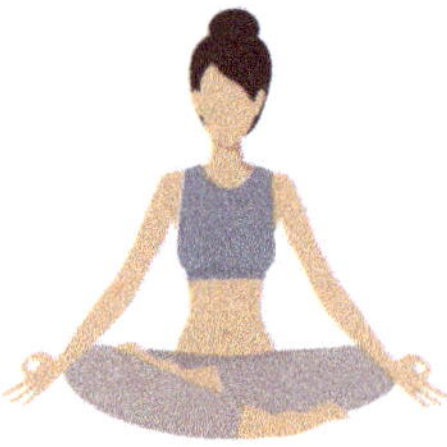

Practice mindfulness

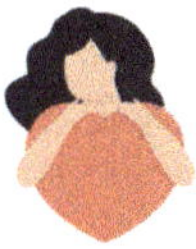

While it can be difficult to break out of negative mental health patterns and develop new routines, there are many things we can do to improve our well-being.

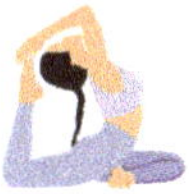

Mindfulness techniques such as meditation, deep-breathing, and yoga can help us become more present and aware of our thoughts and emotions. This can make it easier for us to identify thoughts and beliefs that are keeping us stuck.

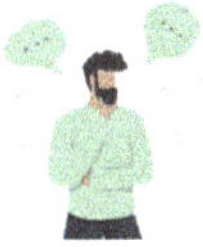

After identifying negative thoughts, we can slowly break free from these patterns and recognize that they are unhelpful by challenging their validity.

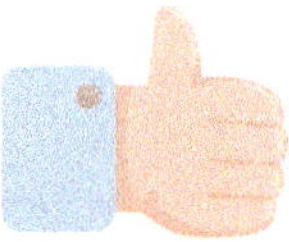

Keep in mind that getting unstuck is a process that takes time and it's okay to take small steps and to be patient with yourself.

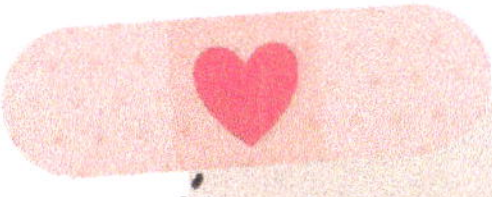

What's one SMALL step you can take right now?

How will you hold yourself accountable?

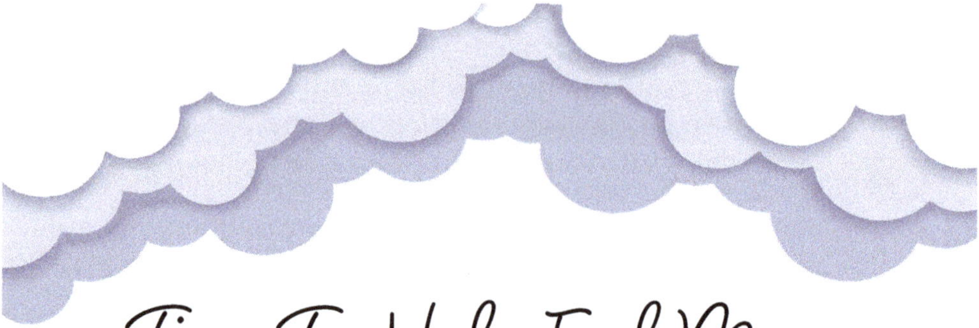

Tips To Help Feel More In Control

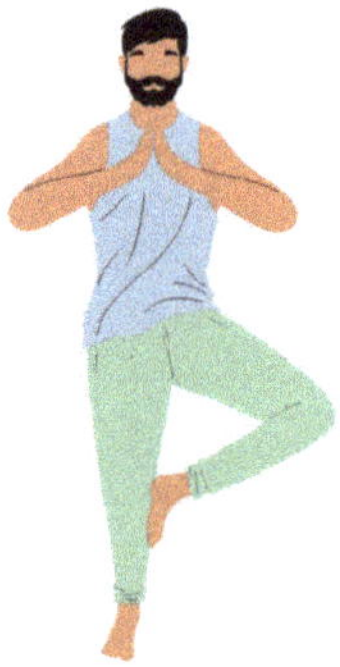

Try a grounding exercise like yoga or meditation

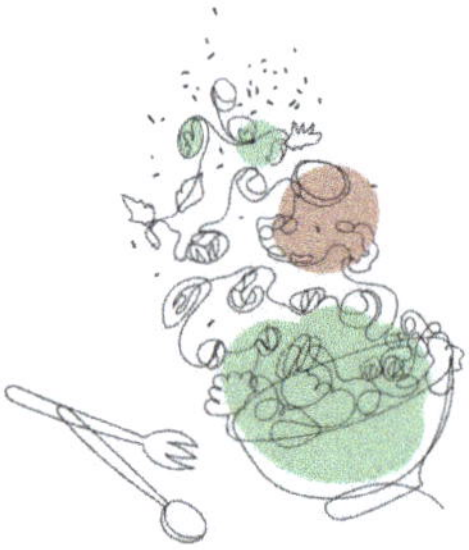

Nourish your body with food and water

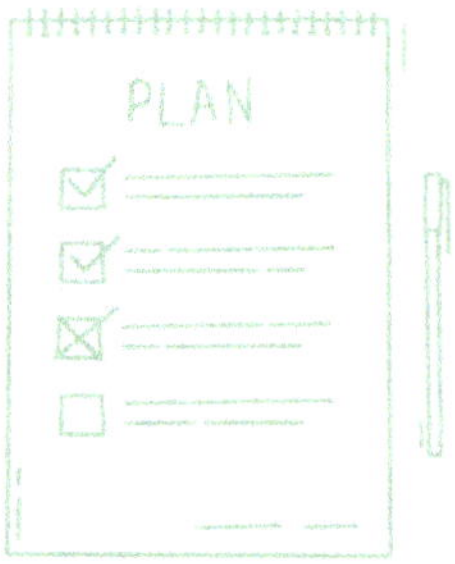

Make a to-do list for the day

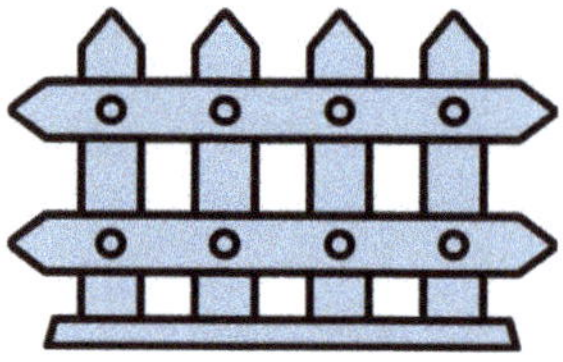

Set boundaries with yourself and others

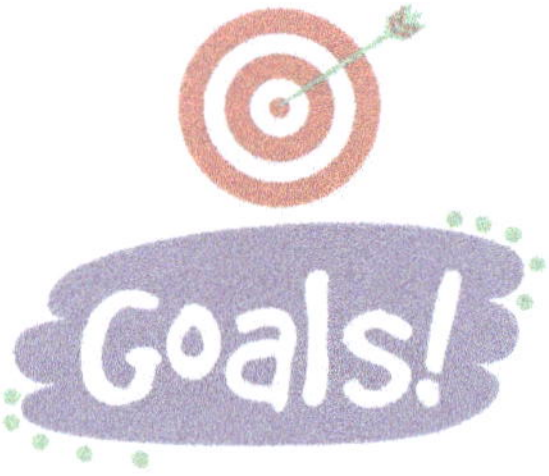

Complete a small task

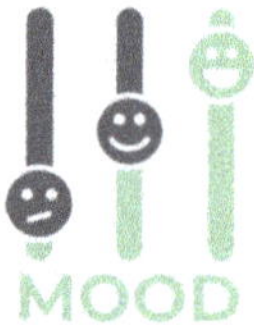

Reflect on your feelings and emotions

Try Tapping

Emotional Freedom Technique (EFT), also known as tapping, focuses on working energy points on the body with your fingertips to release difficult or stuck feelings. To give it a try, choose a point to tap, then fill in the blank with an affirmation (p.147) you can use while you tap.

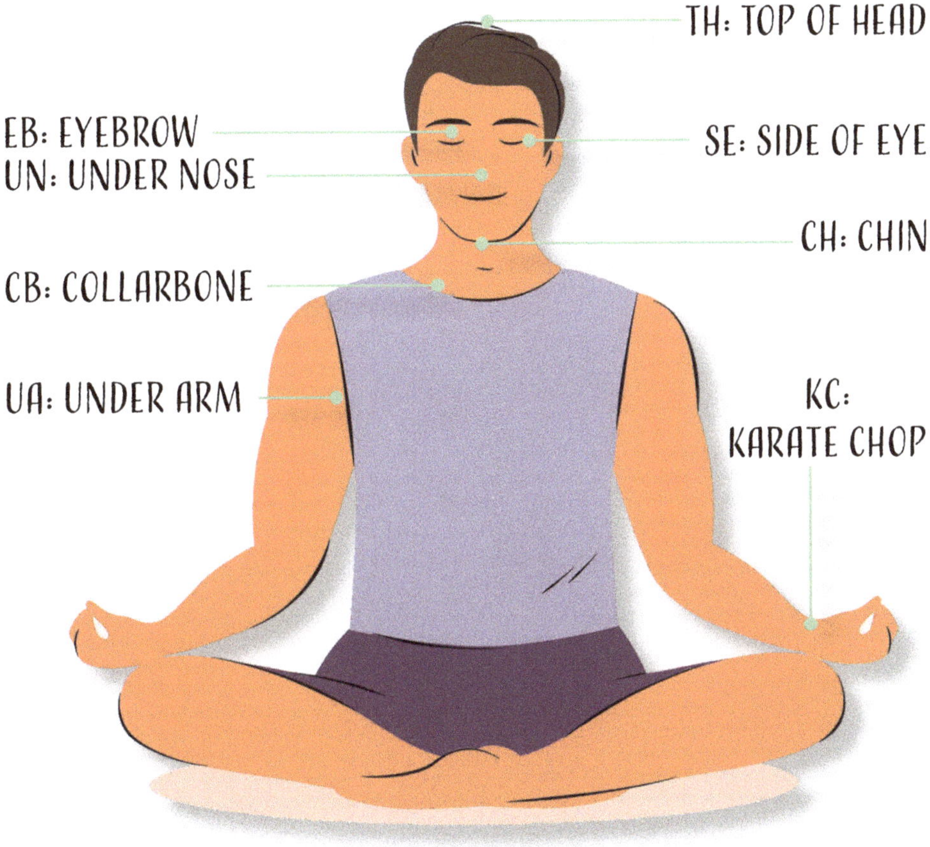

EVEN THOUGH I FEEL ________________, I LOVE AND ACCEPT MYSELF.

Small Encouragements

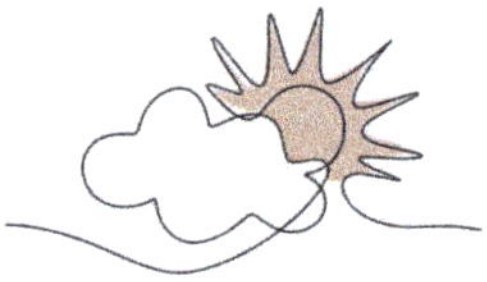

Bad days will not last forever

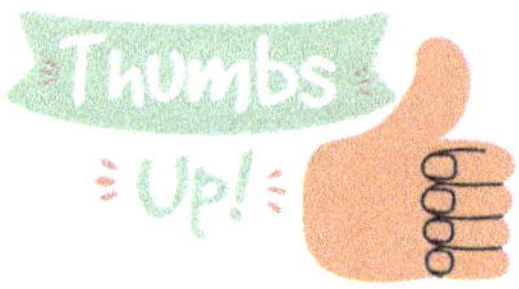

You don't have to be perfect to be worthy

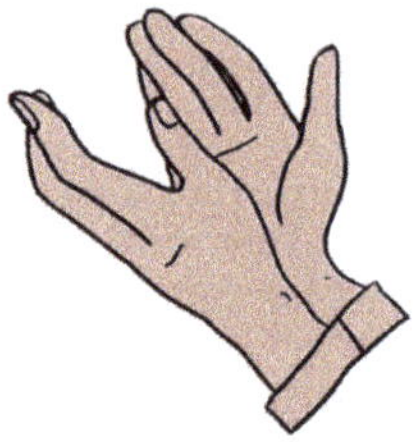

It's okay to start over and try again

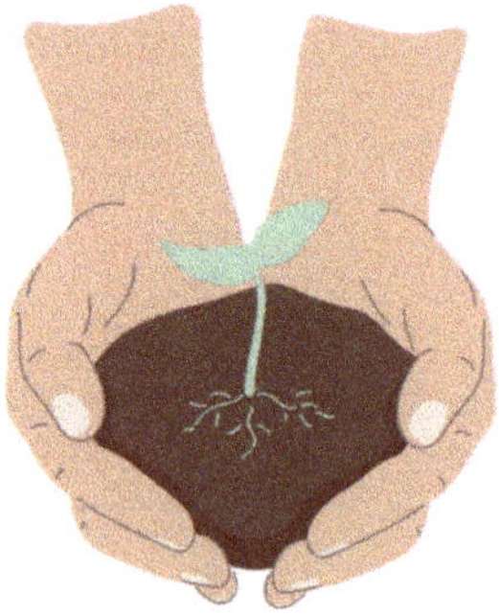

There is something good in each day

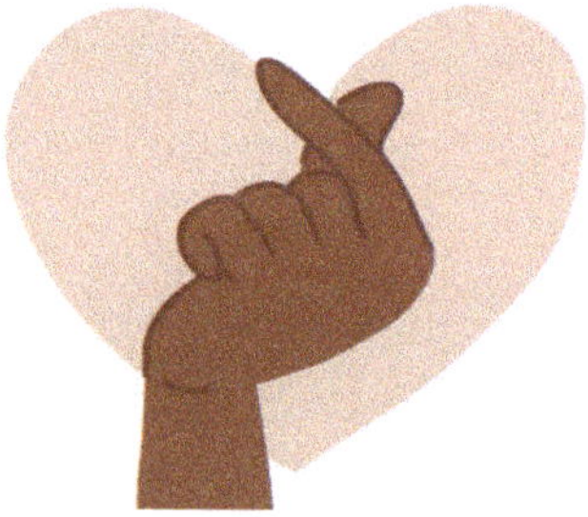

Give yourself grace today

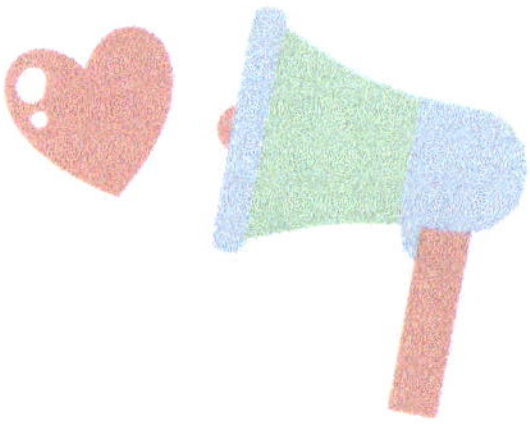

Doing your best is always enough

My solution today to get unstuck will be...

day 12

Asking "What" Questions

"What" Questions allow you to move towards something, keeping you present-focused and able to move into solutions thus finding resolutions. What questions can help you make an action plan to stop anxiety or the fear of the unknown; allowing you to modify and change unwanted behavior patterns and create new habits. (p.336)

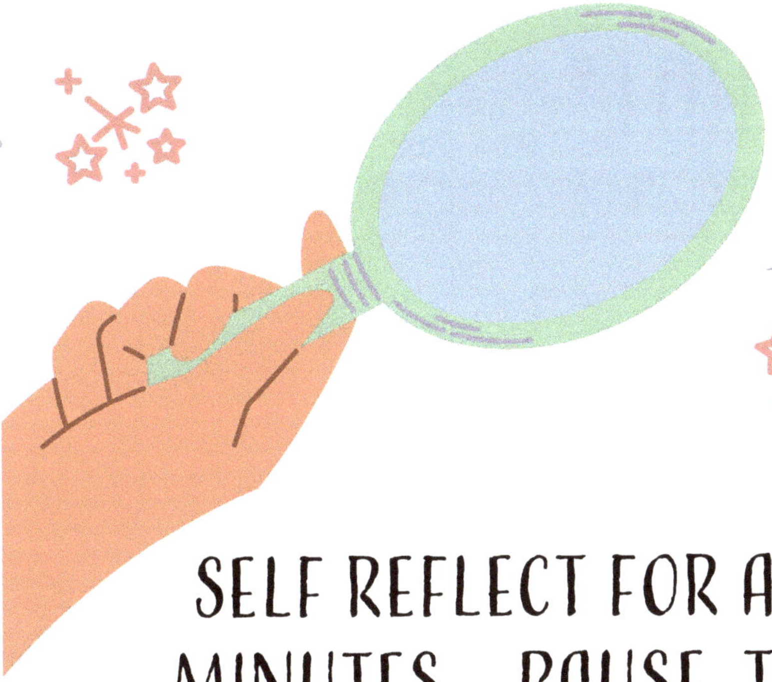

SELF REFLECT FOR A FEW MINUTES... PAUSE, TAKE A BREAK AND CELEBRATE ALL OF YOUR HARD WORK!

JUMP UP AND DANCE TO YOUR FAVORITE SONG!

JUMP UP AND DANCE TO SHAKE IT ALL OUT AND LET IT GO! YOU'VE GOT THIS!

"WHAT" Questions

Ask yourself and write your answers below

WHAT is something my body and mind need?

"WHAT" Questions

Ask yourself and write your answers below

WHAT activities help me recharge?

"WHAT" Questions

Ask yourself and write your answers below

WHAT have I done in similar situations in the past?

"WHAT" Questions

Ask yourself and write your answers below

WHAT can I do that will bring me joy today?

"WHAT" Questions

Ask yourself and write your answers below

Think of a problem that you're struggling with right now. Name it here:

"WHAT" Questions

Ask yourself and write your answers below

WHAT does this solution mean for me right now?

"WHAT" Questions

Ask yourself and write your answers below

WHAT proof do I have that this is fact versus fiction?

"WHAT" Questions

Ask yourself and write your answers below

WHAT is the likelihood of the worst case scenario happening?

day 13

Asking "Why" Questions

"Why" Questions allow you to move into processing by analyzing the past. Why questions are important to help you discover your past thoughts, feelings, behaviors and where you 're getting stuck, by examining your core beliefs. By analyzing your past, you can identify those behaviors that aren't serving you anymore and move into new ways of behaving, thinking, and being. (p.336)

"WHY" Questions

Think of a problem that you're struggling with right now. Name it here:

"WHY" Questions

Ask yourself and write your answers below

WHY do I feel this way?

"WHY" Questions

Ask yourself and write your answers below

WHY am I feeling triggered?

"WHY" Questions

Ask yourself and write your answers below

WHY am I experiencing this thought?

"WHY" Questions

Ask yourself and write your answers below

WHY do I struggle with boundaries?

"WHY" Questions

Ask yourself and write your answers below

WHY do I feel overwhelmed in certain situations?

"WHY" Questions

Ask yourself and write your answers below

WHY do I think this way about myself?

"WHY" Questions

Ask yourself and write your answers below

WHY do I always do this?

"WHY" Questions

Ask yourself and write your answers below

And why does that work (or not work) for me?

day 14

Creating Self-Care

Self-care refers to activities and practices that individuals engage in to promote their physical, mental, emotional and spiritual well-being. Self-care can be an important component of maintaining overall health and preventing stress which can cause burnout. Self-Care activities include: physical self-care, emotional self-care, mental self-care, social self-care, and spiritual self-care. (p.335)

Six Productivity Reminders

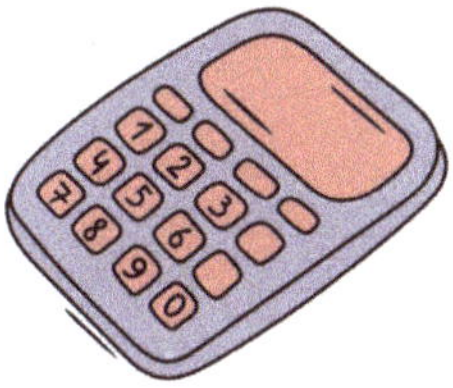

No one is
productive
all the time

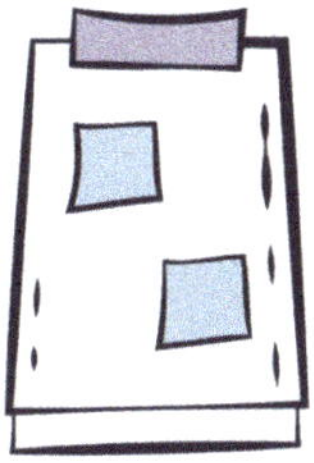

It's okay to
take things at
your own pace

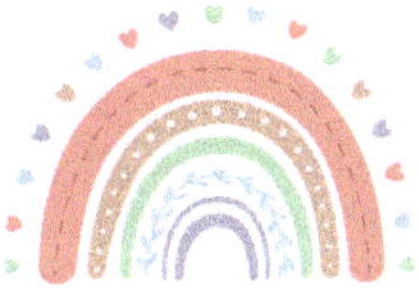

There is much
more to life
than work

Small wins are
still worth
celebrating

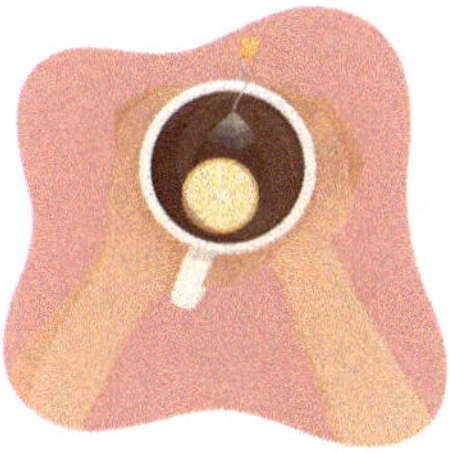

You are
deserving
of breaks

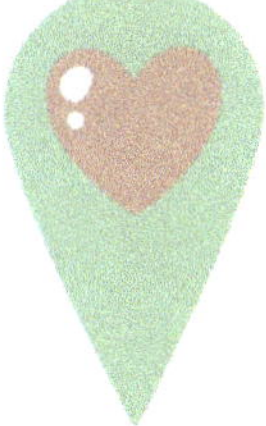

Your best
effort is
enough

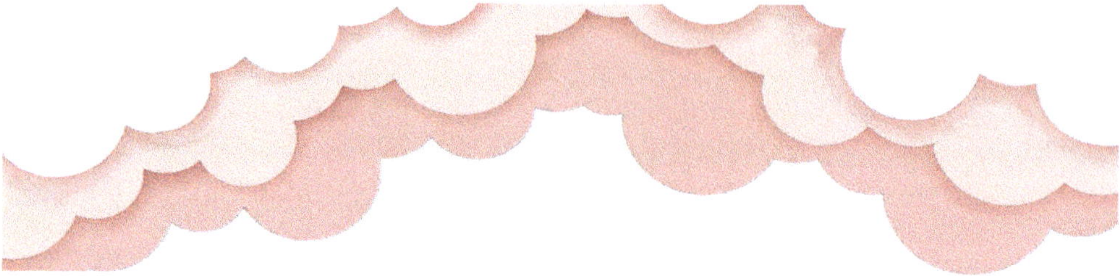

Difficult Acts of Self Care

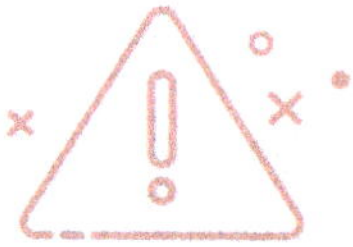

Identifying harmful behaviors and coping skills

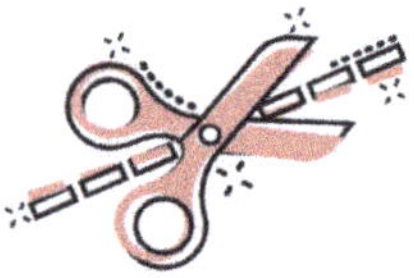

Breaking toxic generational cycles

Learning that your worth is not defined by others

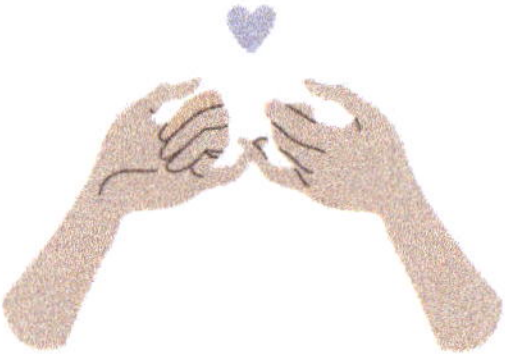

Seeking therapy and support from others

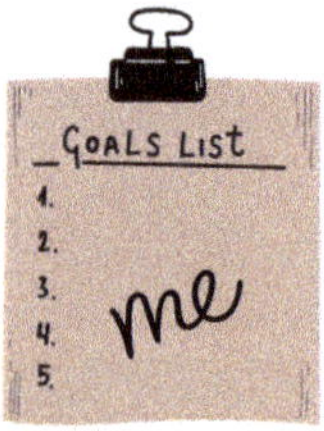

Accepting that it's okay to make yourself a priority

Learning to process feelings in healthy ways

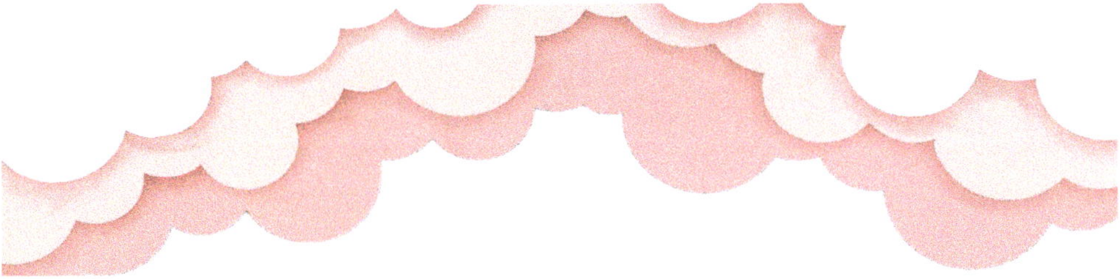

Self care is placing a high value on the wellbeing and happiness of oneself.

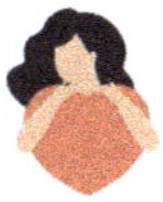

While many forms of self care can be completed in under five minutes, others require more time and commitment.

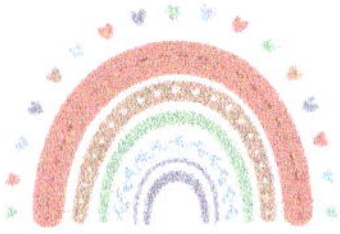

Healing is a process and growth tends to happen over a period of time.

What forms of self care do you find difficult?

I Know I'm Growing When

I am starting to...

I Know I'm Growing When

I am becoming aware of...

I Know I'm Growing When

I am getting better at...

I Know I'm Growing When

I am getting better at...

I Know I'm Growing When

I am breaking negative...

I Know I'm Growing When

I am being more...

I Know I'm Growing When

My mind and body are feeling...

Let's celebrate the AMAZING characteristic you have!

Make a list of 6 of your amazing traits below:

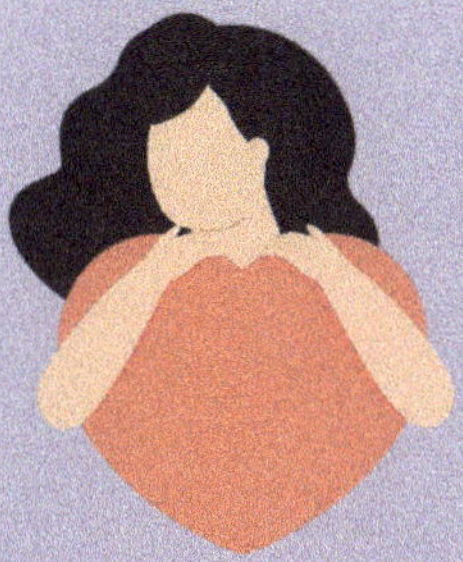

Name the 3 personality traits you want to change about yourself and why. List them below:

day 15

What Are Your Core Beliefs?

Core Beliefs are the deeply held beliefs developed early in life and shaped by our personal experiences, culture, values, spirituality and upbringing that affects what we believe about ourselves, others, and the world. Core beliefs impact our self-confidence and deeply impact how we feel about ourselves in relationship to others. (p.331)

BE KIND
BE KIND
BE KIND
BE KIND

Take All The Self-Love Reminders You Need!

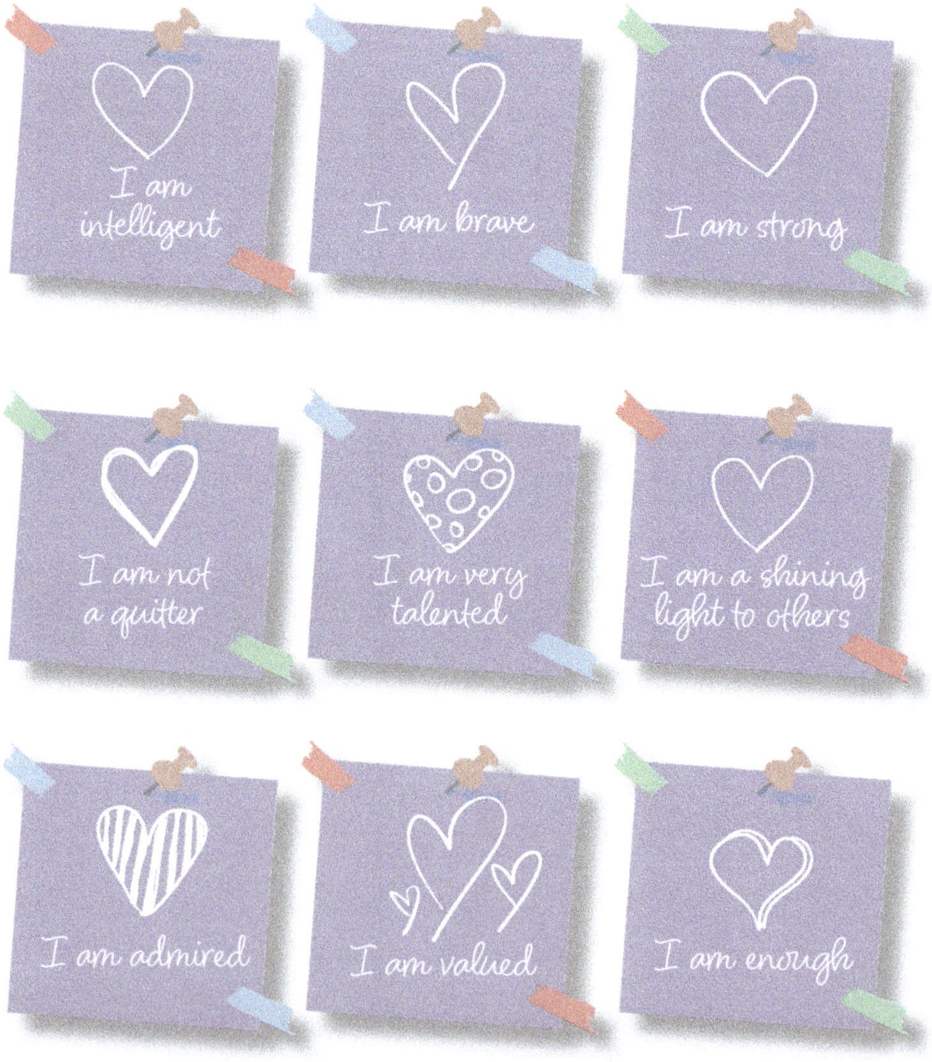

Here I Am Today...

In this moment, I feel...

Where am I getting stuck?

I practice gratitude

yes | no

I get enough sleep

yes | no

I take time to recharge

yes | no

I eat food that makes me feel good

yes | no

I keep my space clean

yes | no

I move my body regularly

yes | no

I take care of my hygiene

yes | no

How Are You Feeling Today?

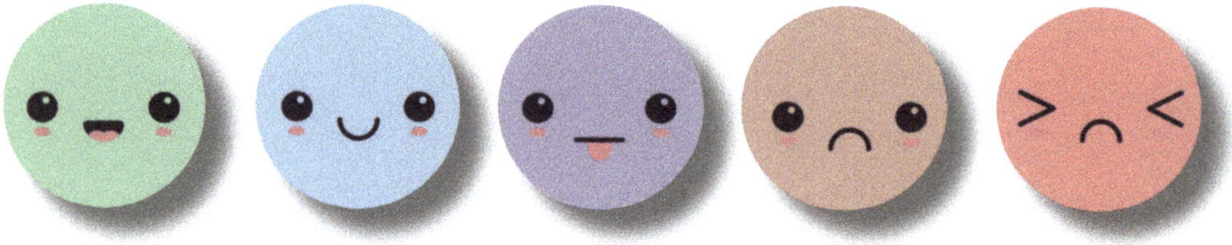

Write down your answer below:

Why are you feeling that in this moment?

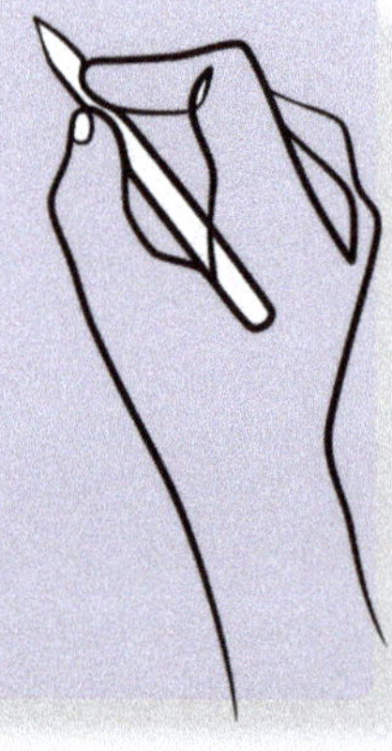

Rating Our Negative Core Beliefs

What do you believe about yourself?

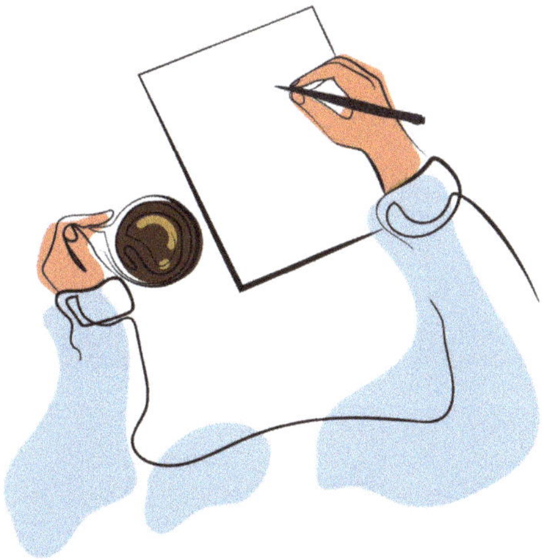

0 NOT AT ALL
1 A LITTLE BIT
2 OFTEN
3 EVERY DAY
4 ALWAYS THERE

- [ ] Unloveable
- [ ] Unworthy
- [ ] an Imposter
- [ ] Embarrassing
- [ ] Not Good Enough
- [ ] Lonely
- [ ] Hurt
- [ ] Abandoned
- [ ] Disgusting
- [ ] Ugly
- [ ] Horrible
- [ ] a Trouble Maker
- [ ] Anger
- [ ] a Perfectionist
- [ ] Fearful
- [ ] Unsafe

What will you commit to for today; write down how you will have more:

Daily Gratitudes

What will you commit to for today; write down how you will have more:

Positive Daily Influencers

What will you commit to for today; write down how you will have more:

Negative Daily Influencers

More Daily Needs

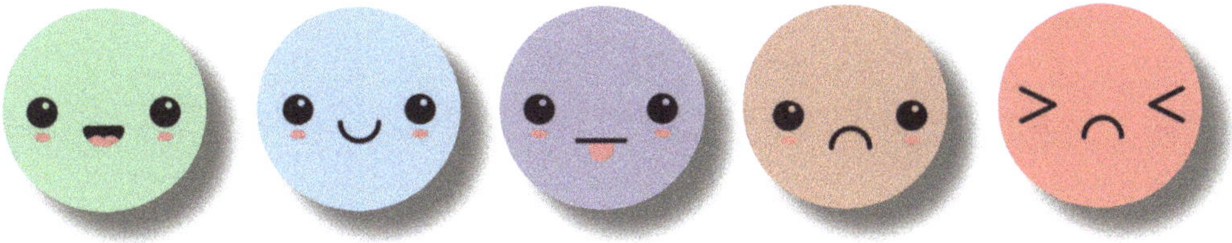

Write down your answer below:

Why are you feeling that in this moment?

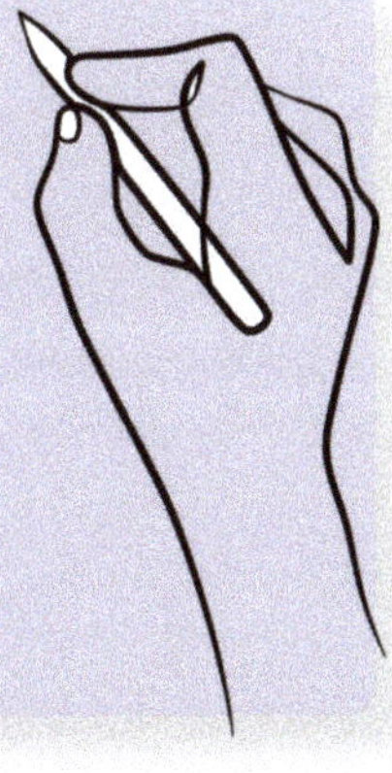

Ways To Self-Regulate

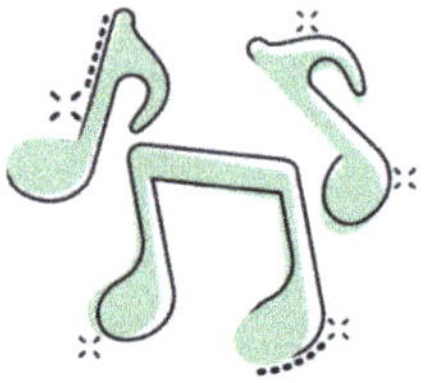

Listen to calming music

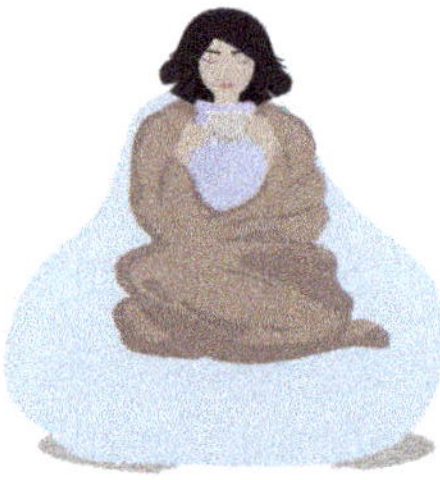

Find a quiet spot to reset

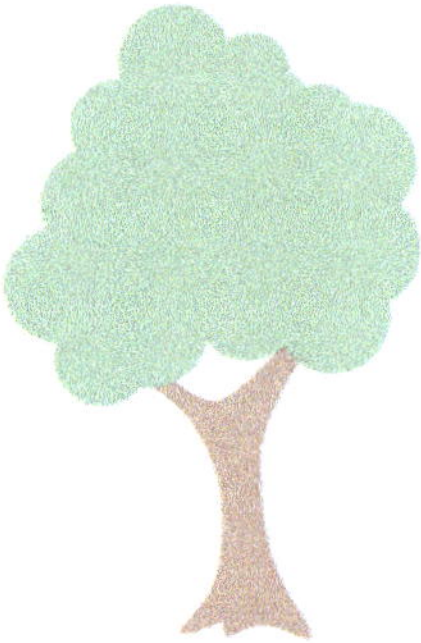

Spend time in nature

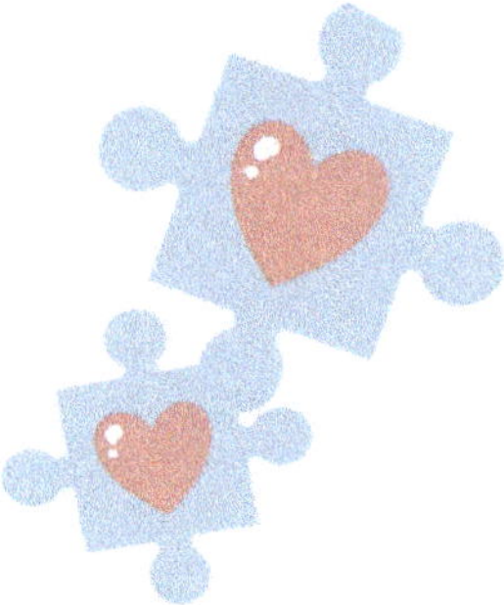

Work on a puzzle or color

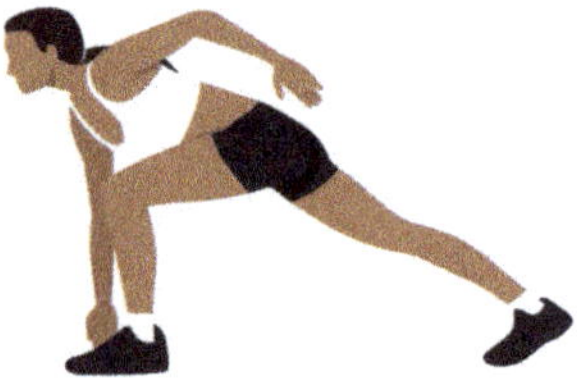

Practice gentle movement

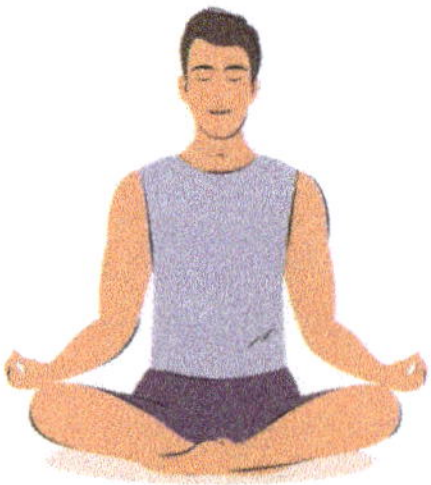

Meditate for 5-10 minutes

Dear

____
(NEGATIVE VOICE NAME),

What I would like from you, _______________
(NEGATIVE VOICE NAME)

is ____

____

____

____

____

____

____

____

____

____!

Sincerely,

____
SIGNATURE

day

16

Redefine Your Emotional Regulation

Emotional Regulation refers to the ability to manage and regulate your own emotions in a healthy and effective way. It involves being able to recognize and understand your emotions, as well as being able to control and modify them in response to different situations. (p.333)

Create A HAPPY Playlist!

The Benefits of Music Include:

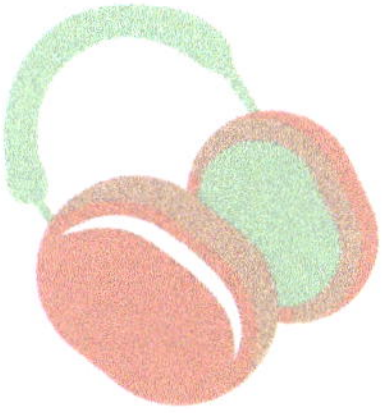

Calms our nervous system and lowers stress

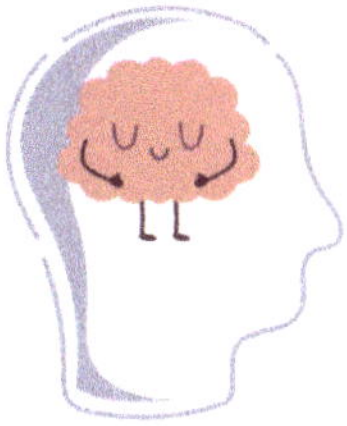

Triggers the release of mood-boosting chemicals

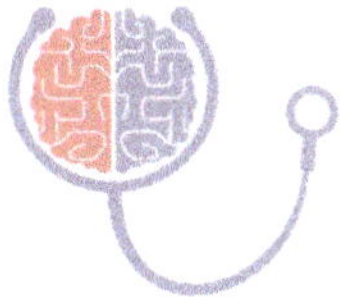

Can improve memory and cognitive function

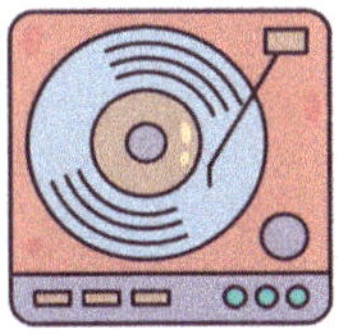

Promotes relaxation and improves sleep

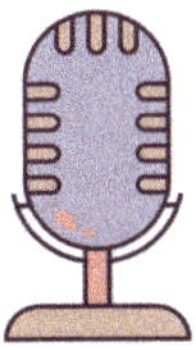

Provides comfort and allows for emotional expression

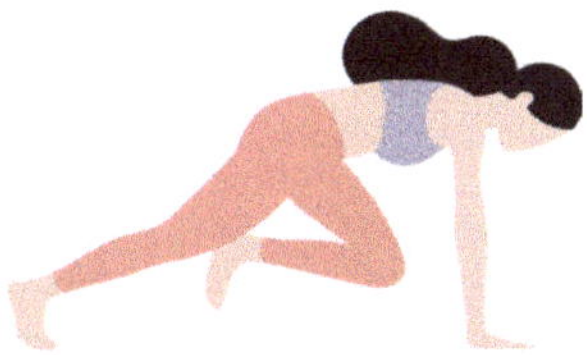

Improves exercise performance

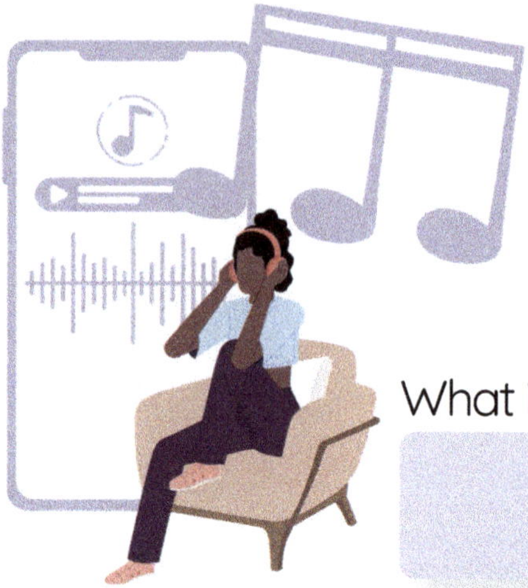

Create your YAY ME Playlist

What is your favorite type of music?

List your favorite songs below!

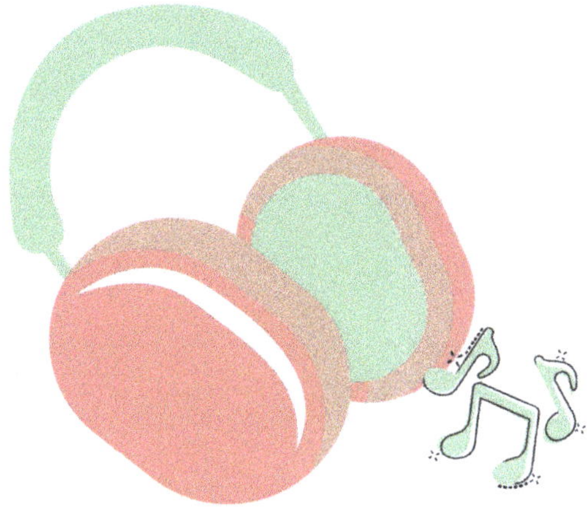

Create your YAY ME Playlist

Create your "I CAN" playlist and list your fav songs here

Create your "UPLIFTING" playlist and list your fav songs here

Ways To Sit With Uncomfortable Emotions

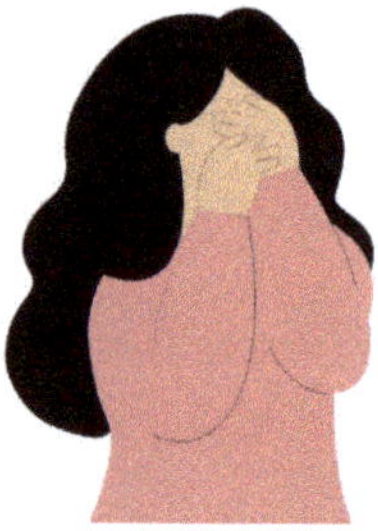

Allow yourself to cry

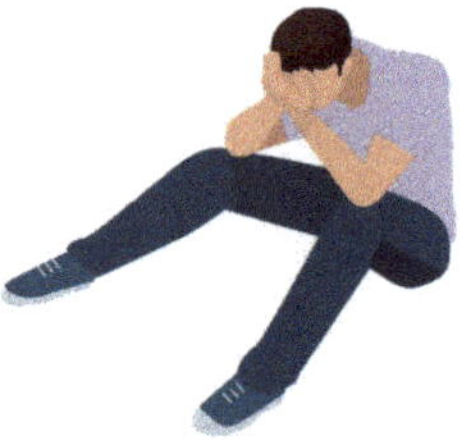

Stay present and mindful

Learn to recognize and identify your feelings

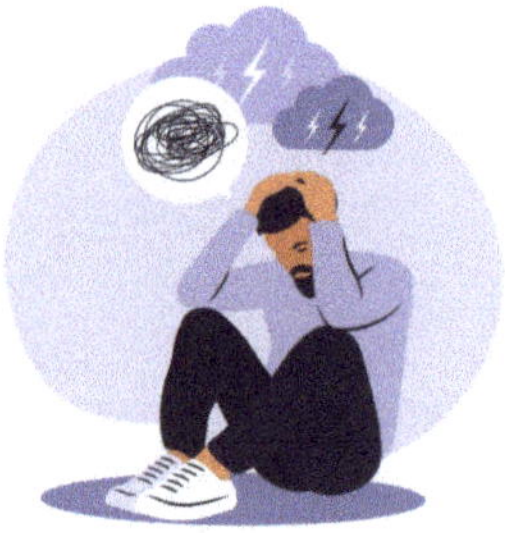

Feel your emotions without judgment

Validate what you are feeling and why you feel it

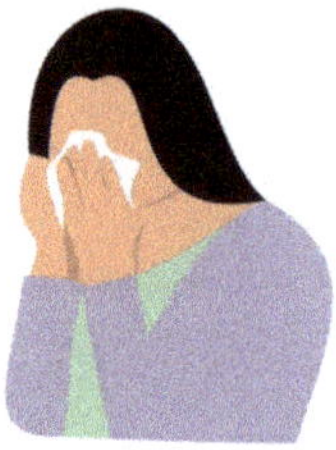

Use coping skills that help you to process the feeling

Progressive Muscle Relaxation

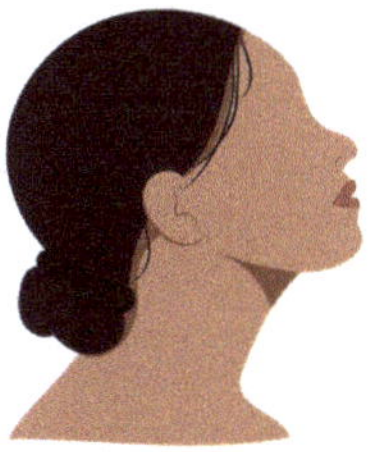

Neck: Nod yes and no, and make slow circles in both direction

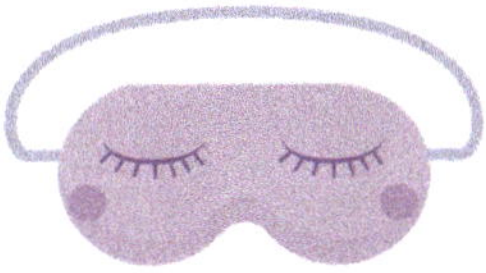

Eyes: Squeeze your eyes tightly shut and then release

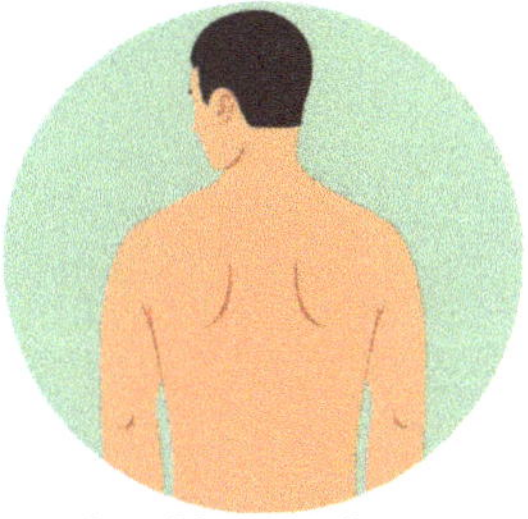

Shoulders: Lift your shoulder blades together, then release them

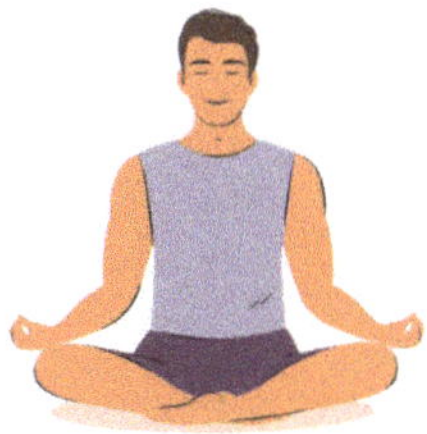

Stomach: Suck in your abdomen gently, then release the tension

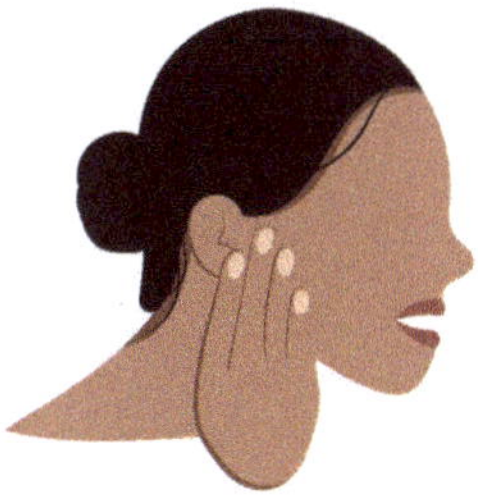

Jaw: Open and close your mouth, then move it left to right

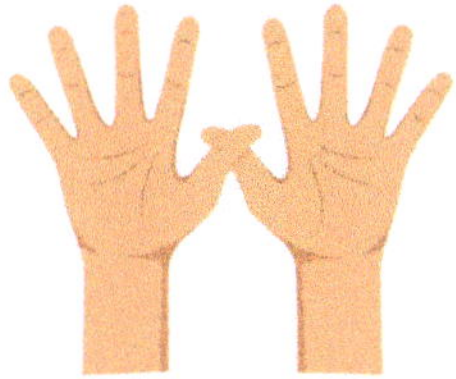

Hands: Curl your fingers into a fist and then release your fingers

How are YOU going to commit to sitting with uncomfortable emotions today?

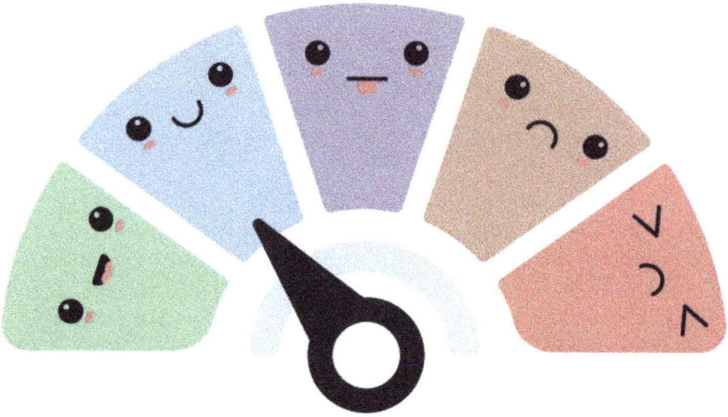

Avoidance

Avoidance is the hallmark of trauma - we use avoidance to escape feelings of fear. How does avoidance work for you and what do you notice about why you tend to be avoidant?

Places I avoid...

Types of people I avoid...

Sounds I avoid...

Memories I avoid think of...

What are some ways that you can work on overcoming your avoidant tendencies?

NOW, let's try some progressive relaxation (p.162) to let that all go!

"Resilience does not mean that we don't react to traumatic and stressful events. Even when we react to particularly stressful or traumatic events, we can still remain resilient."

day 17

Create Emotional Attunement

Emotional Attunement is when you are aware in addition to being responsive to others' needs. This is a fundamentally important skill in interpersonal, romantic and professional relationships. When you're emotionally attuned to others, you're responsive, open, understanding and supportive of the other person's emotional state. (p.332)

Reasons That Crying Can Be Helpful

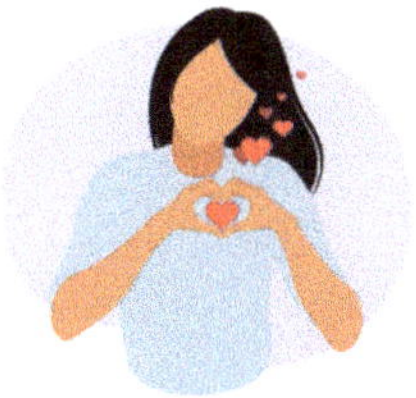

It produces mood-boosting hormones

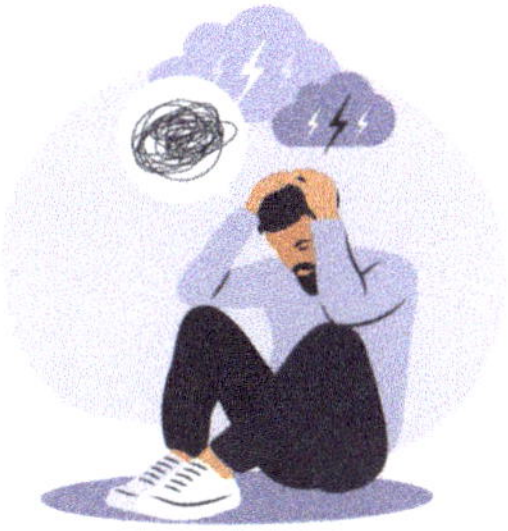

It helps us to release negative emotions

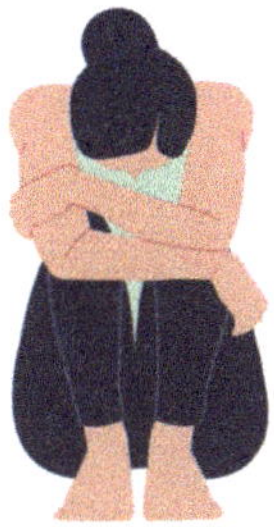

It activates our body's calming response

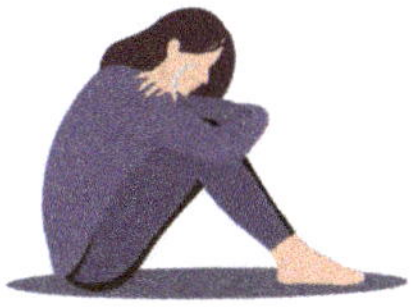

It relieves physical and emotional pain

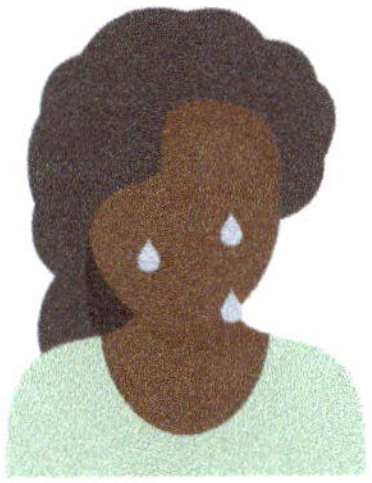

It helps others notice that something is wrong

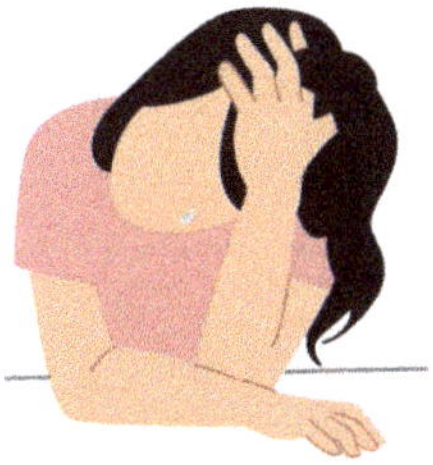

It improves sleep quality

What Our Emotions Tell Us

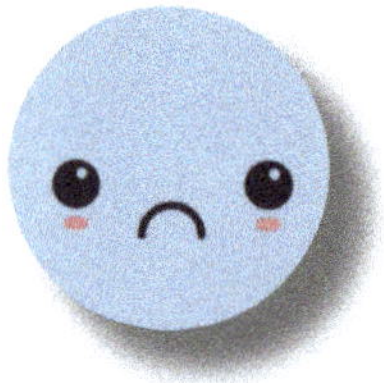

Sadness

Sadness needs to be felt. I need some compassion and love.

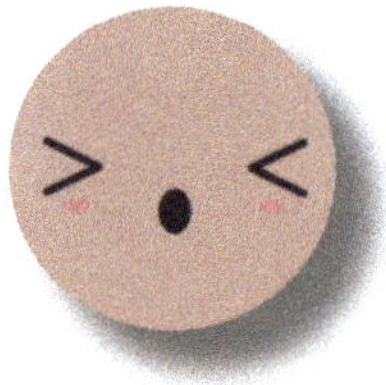

Fear

Fear prepares me for potential danger. I can assess my situation.

Anger

I deserve fairness. I can asssert my needs in a healthy way.

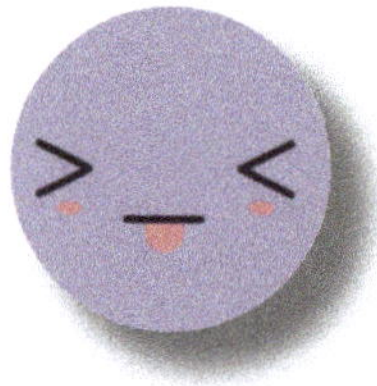

Disgust

The situation does not feel safe. I have the right to say "No."

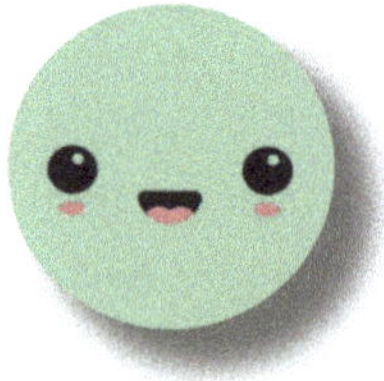

Joy

I am worthy of joy and happiness. I do not need to repress it.

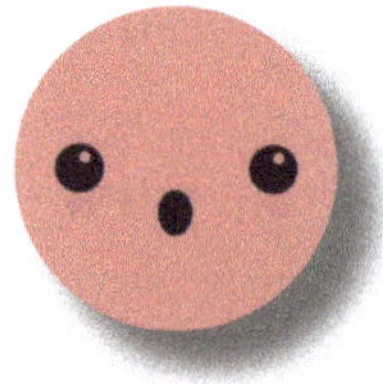

Shame

Shame is unwarranted unworthiness. I am worthy of love.

What is meaningful to me right now to help me with managing my emotions?

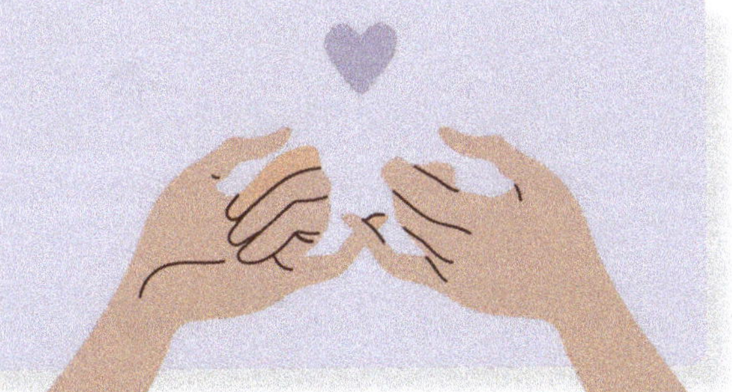

I feel...	I need to...
Overwhelmed	Take a break
Stressed	Focus on relaxation
Anxious	Practice my coping skills
Sad	Be kind towards myself
Angry	Find a positive distraction
Drained	Rest my mind, body, and soul
Broken	Practice self love and compassion

I feel...

I feel...

Speak Up:
POWER WORDS

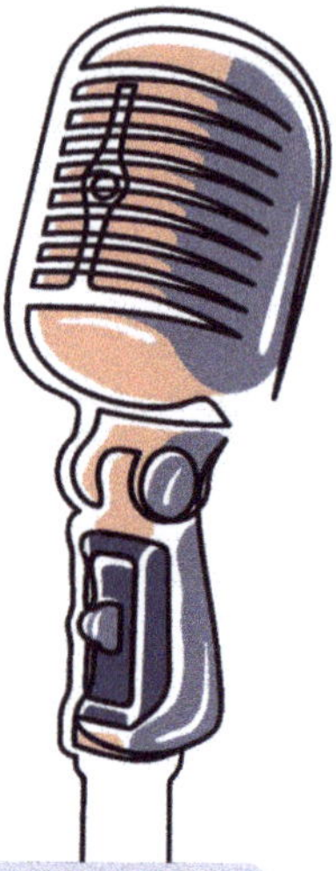

Make a list of your power words (fierce, brilliant, funny) that you can embrace and embody. Practice implementing these power words into your daily life and living.

Get to know your worth

Make a list of all the positive emotions you love about yourself that make you, YOU.

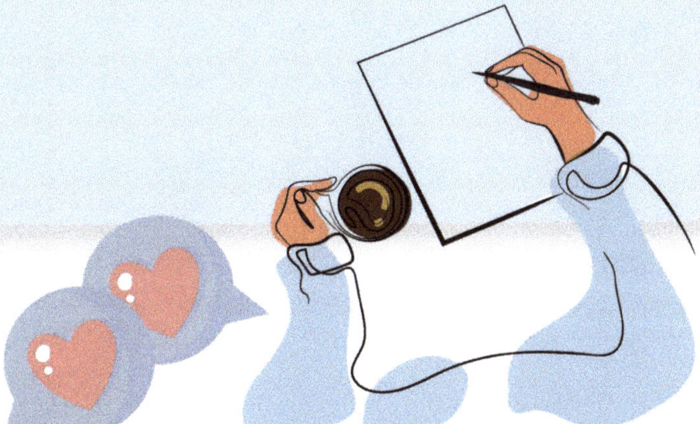

day

18

Self-Love Is Not Selfish

Blame is the act of holding someone responsible for a fault or wrongdoing; an attribution of responsibility for a negative outcome or situation. Blame can be directed towards oneself or others, and it can be harmful depending on the situation. (p.330)

SELF-LOVE
IS NOT SELFISH

Questions To Myself

Ask yourself and write your answers below

WHAT is my main goal in life?

Questions To Myself

Ask yourself and write your answers below

WHAT are my strengths?

Questions To Myself

Ask yourself and write your answers below

HOW will I manifest my perfectly imperfect self today?

Questions To Myself

Ask yourself and write your answers below

WHO matters the most to me?

Questions To Myself

Ask yourself and write your answers below

WHAT am I ashamed of?

Questions To Myself

Ask yourself and write your answers below

WHAT do I like to do for fun?

day 19

Let's Meditate

Perfectionism is a personality trait characterized by the tendency to set extremely high standards for oneself and others, while striving for flawlessness and excellence in all areas of life. Perfectionists often have a strong need for control, and may be highly critical of themselves and others when those standards are not met. Perfectionism can become problematic when it leads to unrealistic expectations, excessive self-criticism, and the belief that things can only be done a certain way. (p.334)

"If I make one small change a day, I will make a lifestyle change which becomes sustainable."

Try this meditation while you're doing your morning wake up and nightly before sleep routine to help you create an imperfect mindset.

While looking in the bathroom mirror, repeat the following:

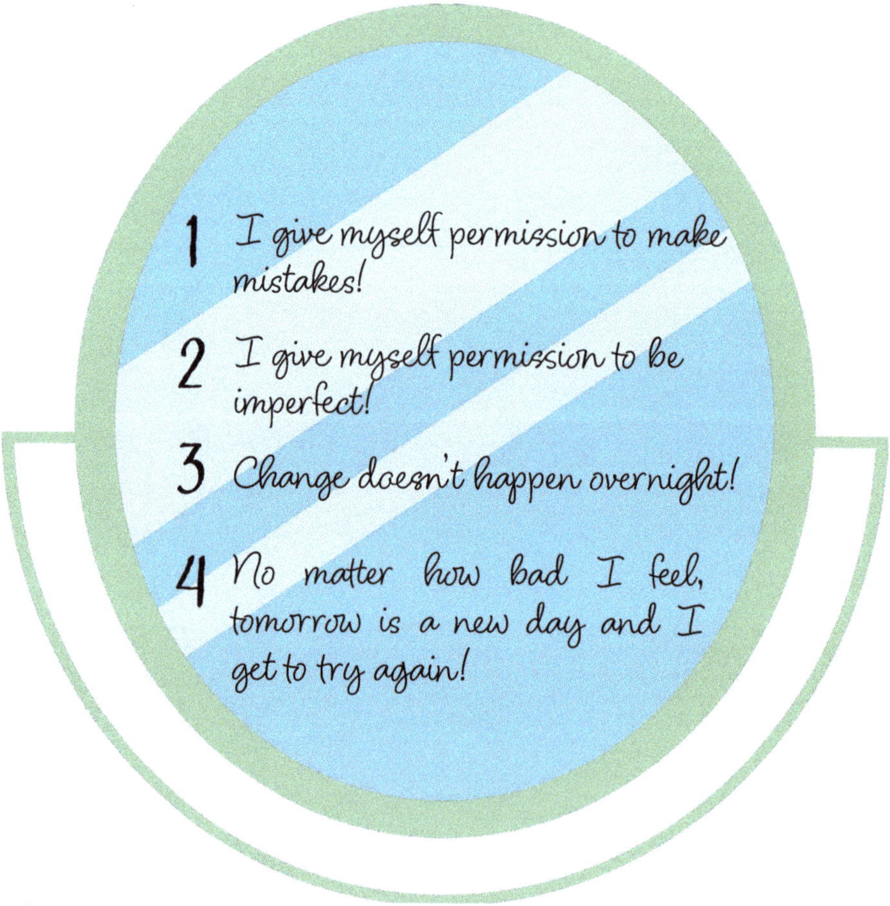

I AM PERFECTLY IMPERFECT

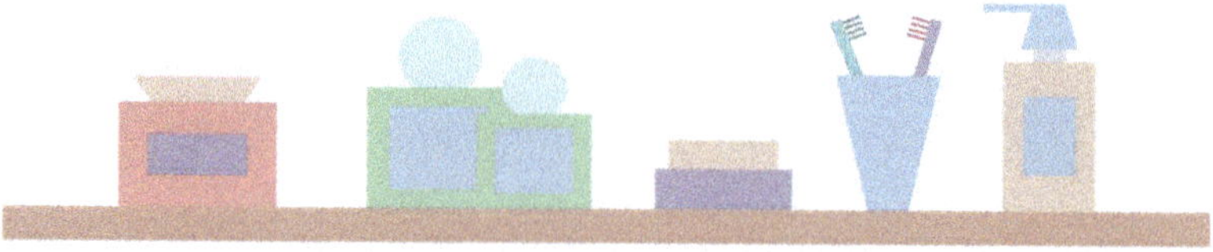

Perfectionism Looks Like...

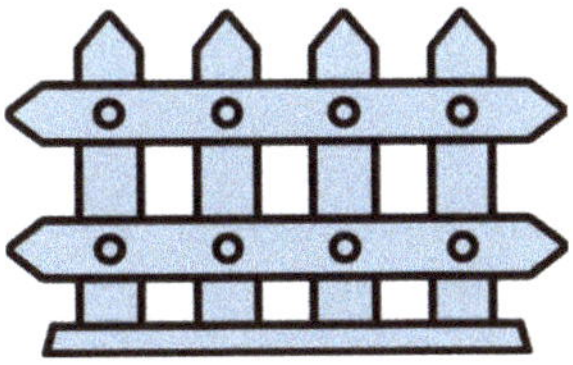

Lack of healthy boundaries

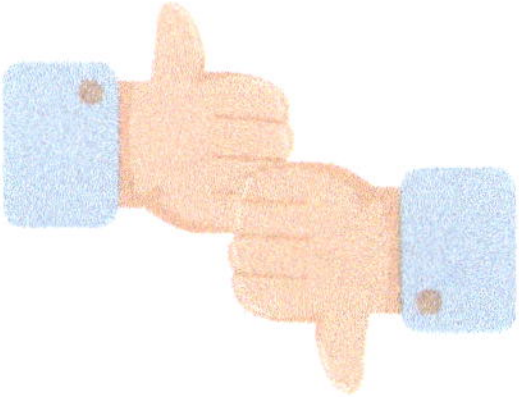

Extreme overachieving or underachieving

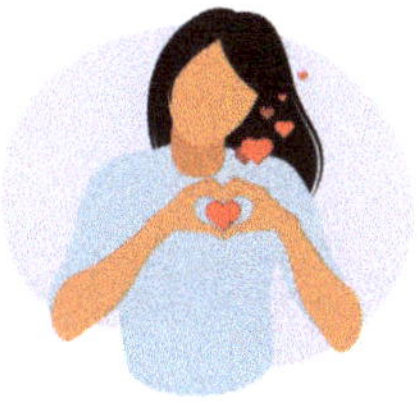

Lack of self-compassion, and self-love

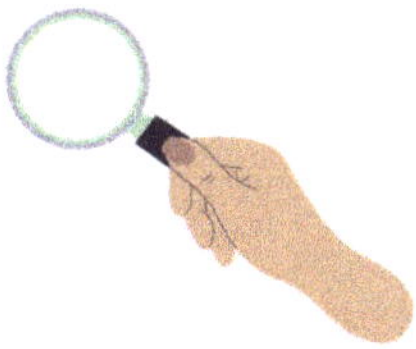

Never being satisfied with self and others

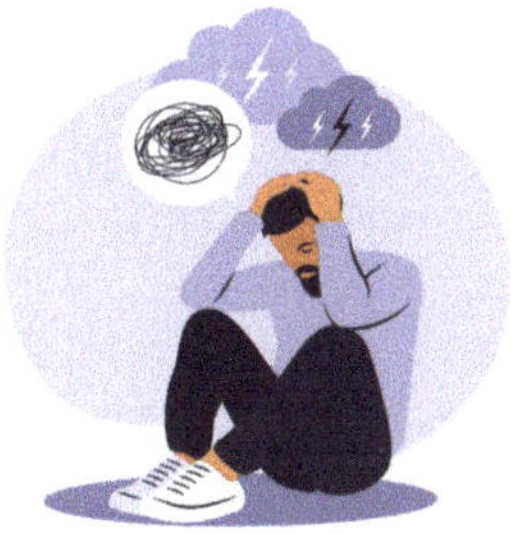

Self-destructive behaviors

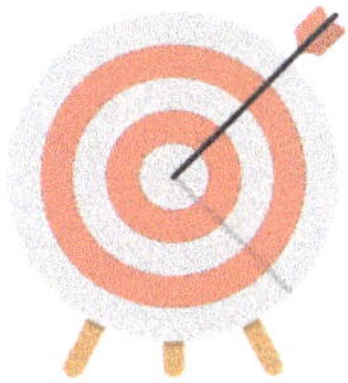

Unrealistic goals and expectations

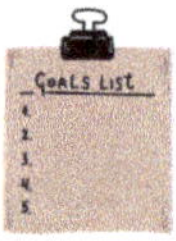

A perfectionist is someone who strives to be perfect.

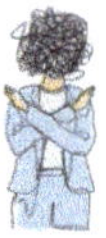

People who are perfectionists tend to have unrealistic expectations for themselves and others, and find it frustrating when these expectations are not met.

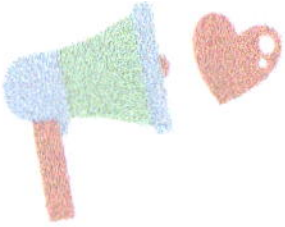

In addition, perfectionists are very hard on themselves and struggle to accept mistakes or express self compassion.

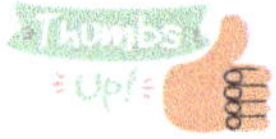

This self criticism also plays into successes as perfectionists are unlikely to celebrate themselves when they do something well because of their very high standards.

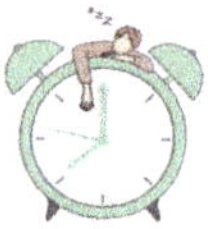

Some ways to reduce perfectionism are to practice regular acts of kindness towards yourself, set realistic expectations, establish a time limit for tasks, and challenge your inner critic.

In what ways have your behaviors turned you into a perfectionist?

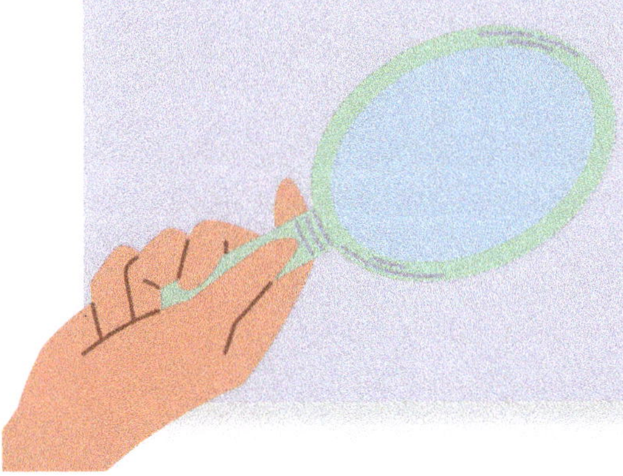

What are some realistic goals that you can set?

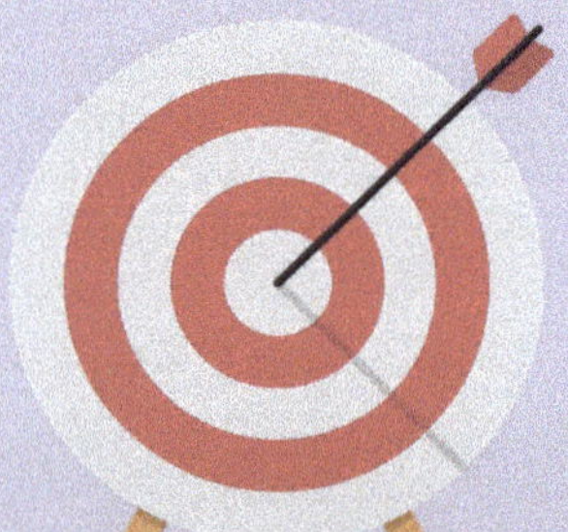

Reframing The "What Ifs"

How can you reframe your thoughts?

What if I go and do not have fun?	→	What if I have a great time?
What if I fail?	→	What if I do okay?
What if they laugh at me?	→	What if they'll be my new friends?
What if I never achieve this goal?	→	What if trying my best is good enough?
What if I make a mistake?	→	What if we all make mistakes?

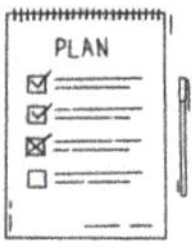

One way to reframe "what ifs" is to focus on the present moment. Instead of worrying about what might happen in the future, remind yourself of the things you can control in the present.

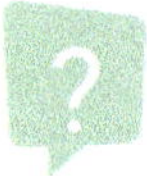

This can help you to focus on the things you can do to prepare for potential challenges, rather than focusing on worst-case scenarios.

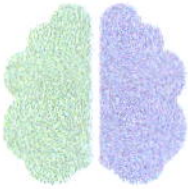

Another way to reframe "what ifs" is to consider the likelihood of the event actually happening.

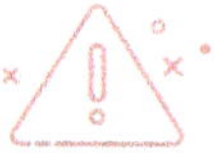

Many "what ifs" are based on unlikely events, and by considering the actual likelihood of the event, we can put our worries into perspective and release ourselves from the anxiety.

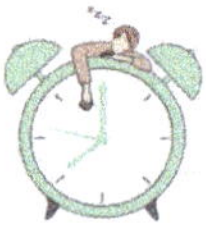

Reframing "what ifs" can take time, but it's a valuable skill to develop for managing anxiety and uncertainty in our lives. As we take control of our thoughts and focus on the present moment, we can reduce worry and improve our mental well-being.

What thoughts can you reframe?

Perfectly Imperfect

What's your TOP 10 Perfectly Imperfect challenges?

1

2

3

4

5

6

7

8

9

10

Try Something New This Month

What stops you from taking a mental health day? What are you afraid of? How can you commit to giving yourself a much needed break? Put a date on the calendar and hold yourself accountable.

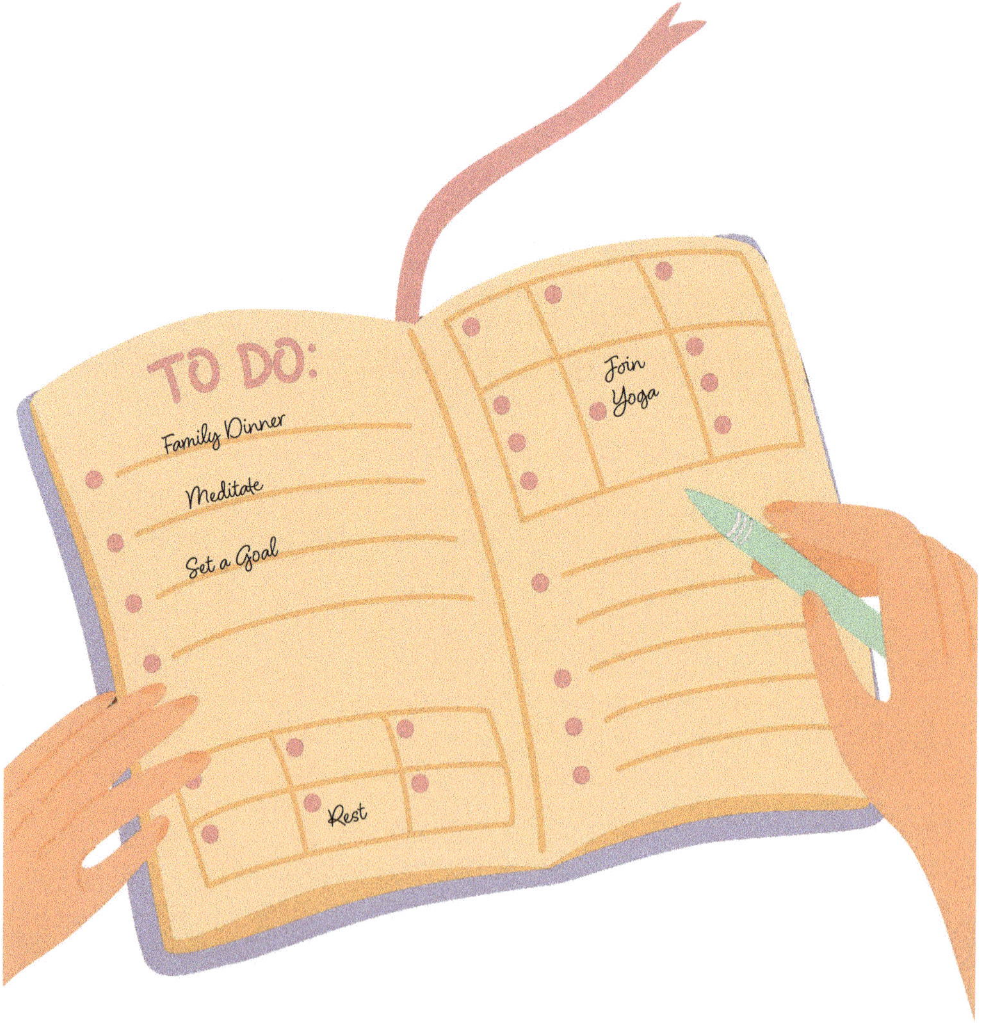

"In times of stress, the best thing we can do for each other is to listen with our ears and our hearts and to be assured that our questions are just as important as our answers."

-Fred Rogers

day 20

Creating A Gratitude Practice

Gratitude refers to a feeling of appreciation, thankfulness, or recognition for the good things in one's life. It involves acknowledging and being mindful of the positive aspects of one's experiences, relationships, and circumstances, rather than focusing on the negative or lacking aspects. Gratitude can be directed towards oneself, others, or a higher power or source. (p.333)

Ways To Express Self-Love

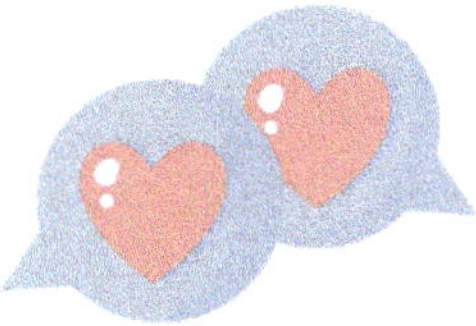

Give yourself a compliment

Keep a gratitude journal

Cut off negative self-talk

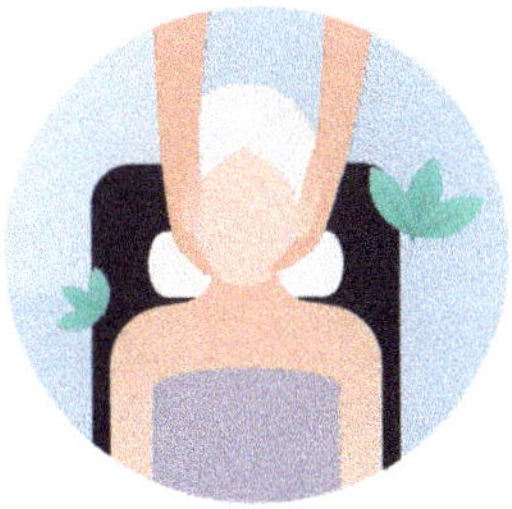

Get a relaxing massage

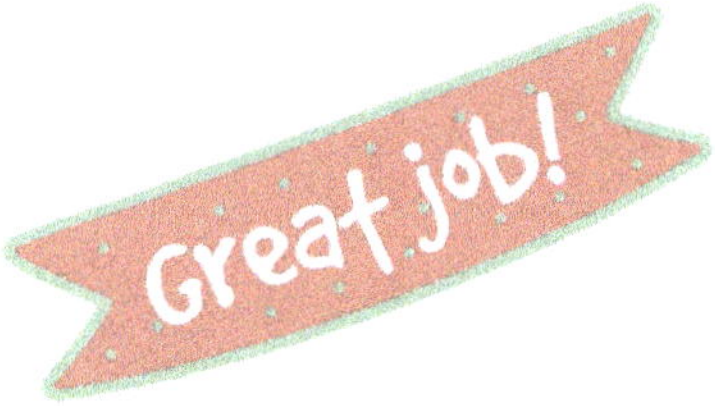

Celebrate small wins

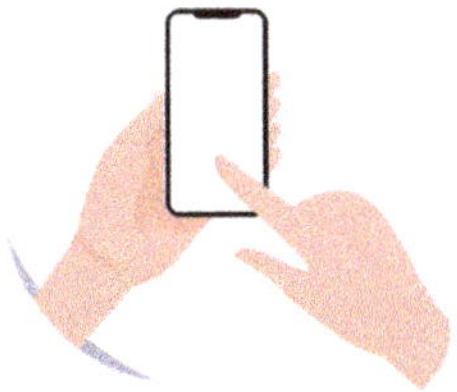

Limit time on social media

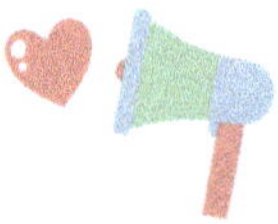

The act of practicing self-love involves caring for oneself and engaging in activities that promote positive well-being.

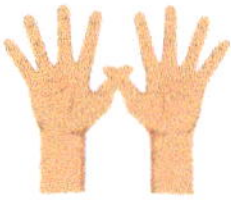

Nurturing your body, your mind, your emotions, and your spirit can help boost your mood and enhance your sense of well-being naturally.

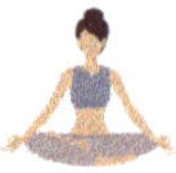

Furthermore, many of these activities don't require a lot of time or effort to benefit from them.

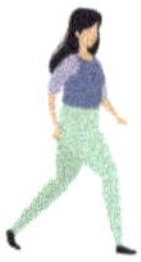

It can be as simple as lighting a scented candle during dinner, picking up your favorite drink on the way to work, or even taking a walk around the block.

Make a list of some ideas that will promote your positive well-being. Write it down here:

Mental Health Check-in

Share below how you're feeling with an emoji.
Circle the emoji that best fits your mood right now.

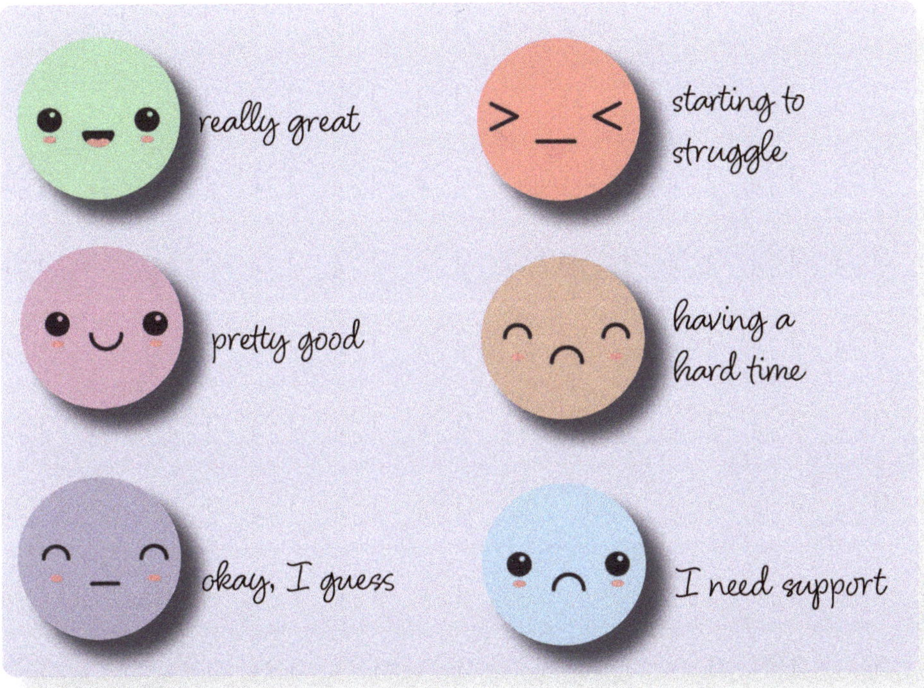

Check-in expert mode: keep a weekly log of your mood every morning and every night. See what patterns you notice. On the low days, try an energy givers activity (p.96).

Why are you feeling this way?

Types of Self-Love

- Stress management
- Self-compassion
- Kindness towards others

- Moving your body
- Eating nutritious food
- Getting enough sleep

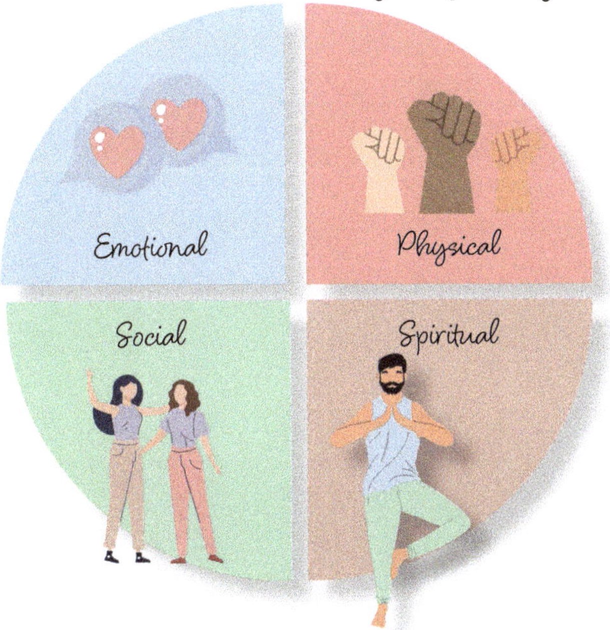

- Setting boundaries
- Positive social media influence
- Having a strong support system

- Meditation and mindfulness
- Journaling
- Spending time in nature

My Self-Love Activities

Pick out a few self-love activities and try them this week!
What are you willing to try? Write them down below:

Try writing a gratitude letter:

Who are you grateful for?

Now, write a letter to one of the people you are grateful for; guided by the following steps. Write as if you are speaking to this person directly ("Dear ___").

1. Don't worry about grammar or spelling.
2. Describe in specific terms what this person did, why you are grateful to this person, and how this persons behavior affected your life. Try to be as concrete as possible.
3. Describe what you are doing in your life now and how you often remember their efforts.
4. Try to keep your letter to roughly one page (around 300 words).

"Whatever we are waiting for—peace of mind, contentment, grace, the inner awareness of simple abundance—it will surely come to us, but only when we are ready to receive it with an open and grateful heart."

– Sarah Ban Breathnach

day 21

What Are Your Values?

Values are the beliefs, principles, and ideals that are important to you. They are the fundamental concepts and standards that guide your behavior, decision-making, and interactions with others. Values can be influenced by a variety of factors, such as culture, religion, personal experiences, and social conditioning. (p.336)

if you're feeling

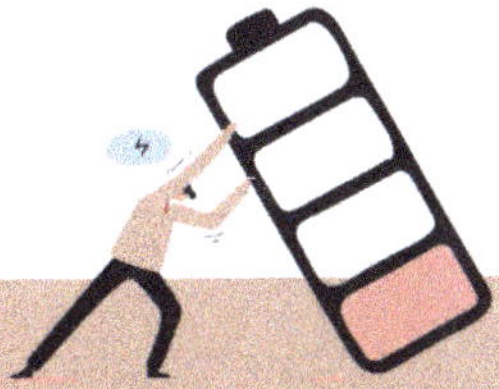

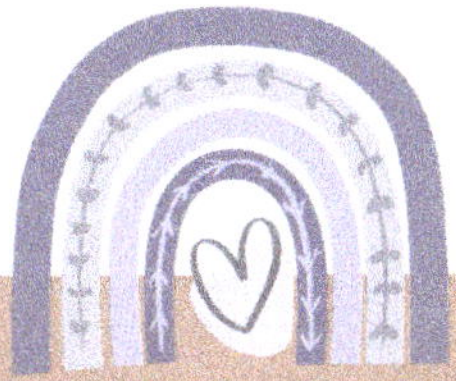

Overwhelmed → Journal

Anxious → Meditate

Burnt out → Walk outside

Sad → Call a friend

Angry → Breathing exercises

It's Okay To Outgrow

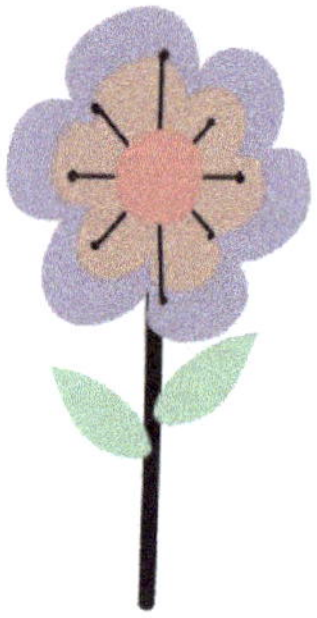

Who you thought you were

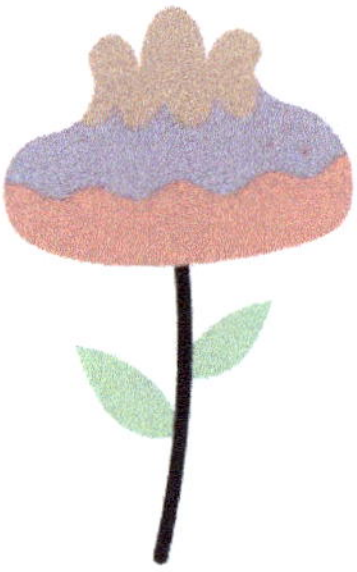

Relationships' and friendships

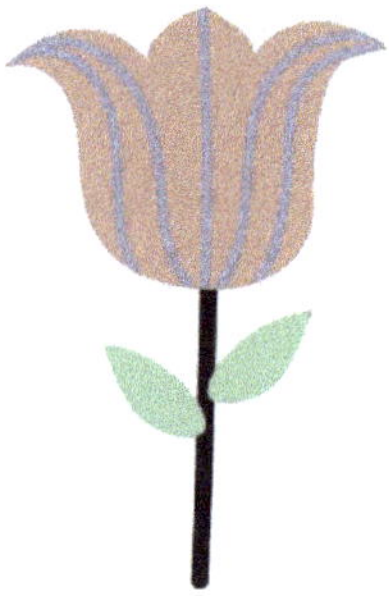

Dreams and goals you had

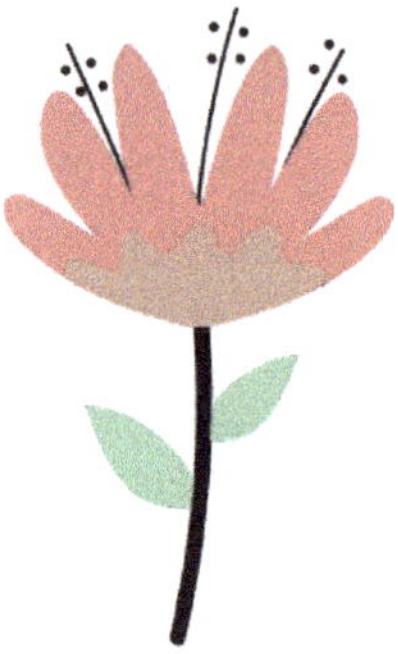

Needing approval from others

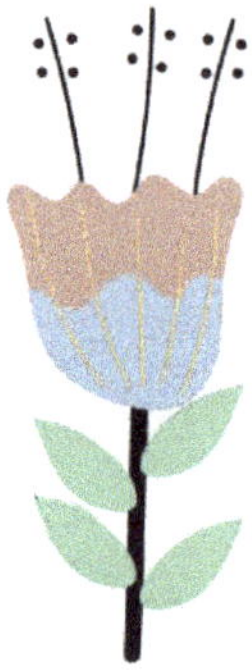

Your old ways of thinking

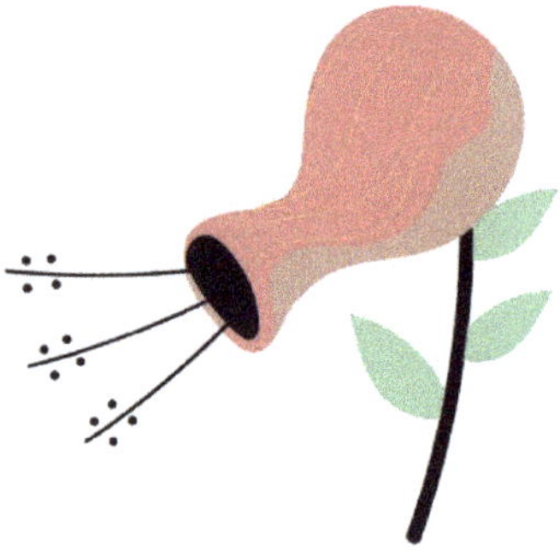

Habits and coping mechanisms

It's okay to outgrow the old version of ourselves.

It's okay to let go of old interests, passions, and hobbies to pursue new ones that bring you joy.

It's okay to outgrow relationships and habits that are unhealthy or do not serve us.

It's okay if you have grown and are no longer the same person you used to be.

What are some things you've outgrown?

Personal Values Bingo Experiment

This bingo game is designed to help you identify the values which can be essential to you. Put a STAR on any of the values below that apply to you.

Justice	Careful	Honesty	Fairness	Merit
Optimism	Mastery	Ambitious	Insight	Clarity
Ability	Wisdom	Grace	Integrity	Resilient
Loyalty	Humility	Efficient	Power	Respect
Control	Ethics	Empathy	Fluency	Balance

Personal Values Bingo Experiment

Circle any of the values below that you want to cultivate in your life.

Justice	Careful	Honesty	Fairness	Merit
Optimism	Mastery	Ambitious	Insight	Clarity
Ability	Wisdom	Grace	Integrity	Resilient
Loyalty	Humility	Efficient	Power	Respect
Control	Ethics	Empathy	Fluency	Balance

How are you going to do more to cultivate the values you desire?

Self-Love Solo Date Ideas

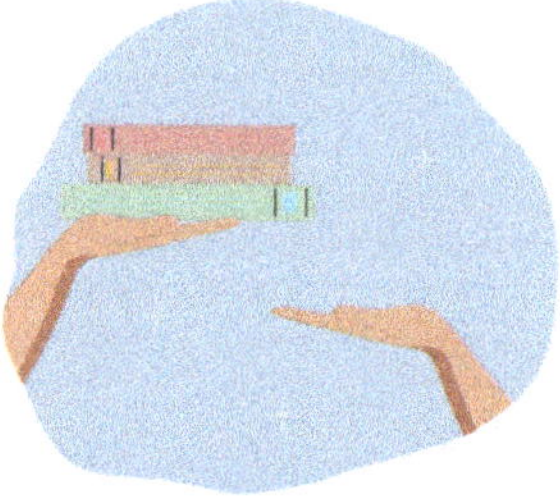

Visit a library

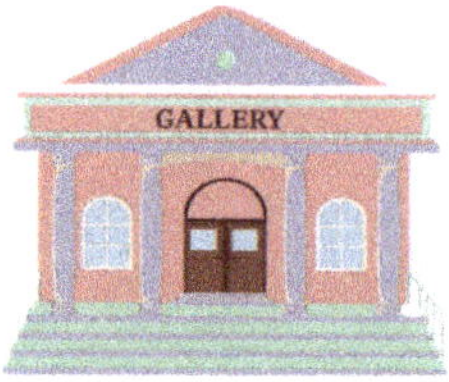

Spend day at a museum

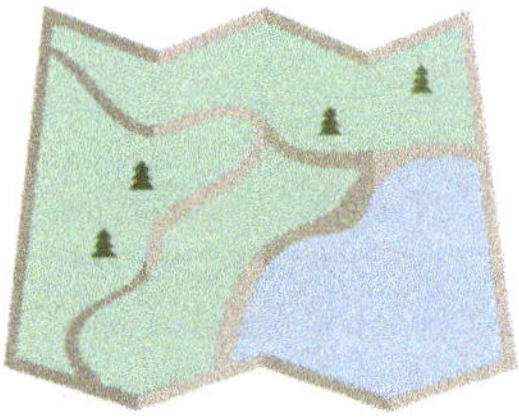

Spend the day in nature

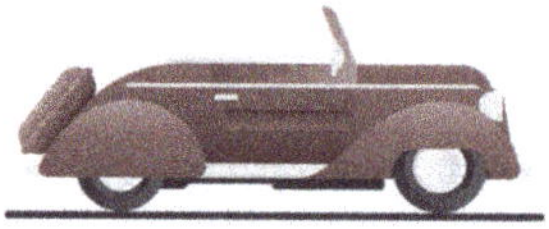

Go for a long drive

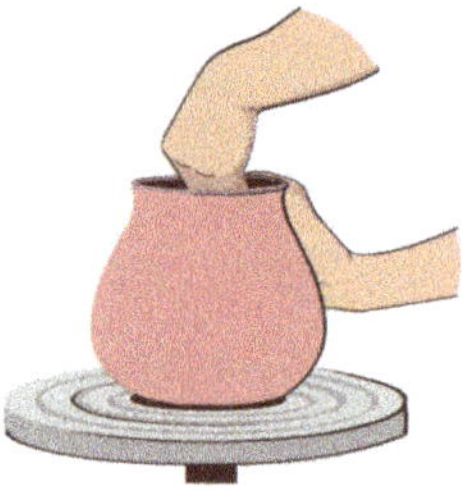

Go to a pottery workshop

Plan a Date With Yourself

Where will you go?

What will you do?

What will you wear?

What will you eat?

How will you get there?

How long will you need?

What are your expectations?

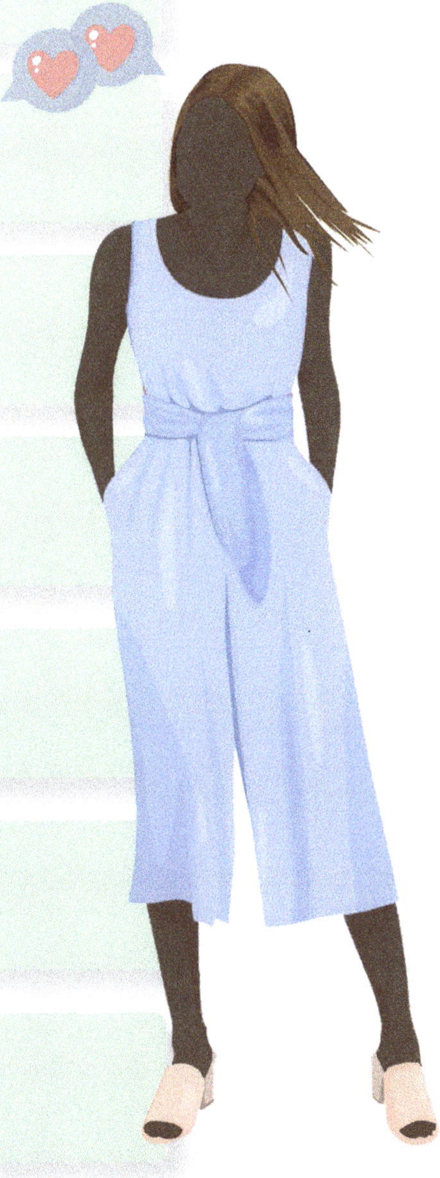

day 22

Connect With Yourself

Connection is a sense of belonging and closeness which consists of the various relationships to others, experiences, thoughts,emotions and behaviors that we form throughout lives. Our interconnectedness to ourselves and others allows us to feel fulfilled and loved. (p.331)

How do you connect with yourself?

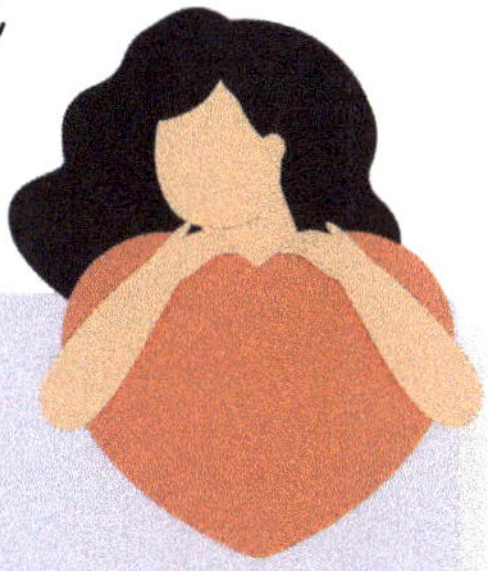

Signs That You May Be Disconnected From Yourself

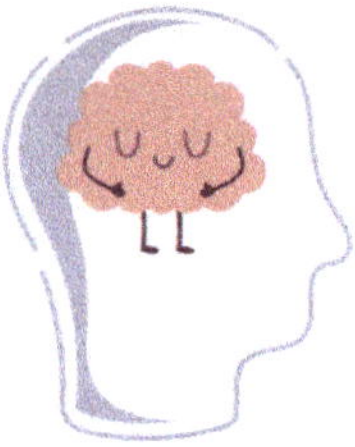

It's hard to identify what brings you joy

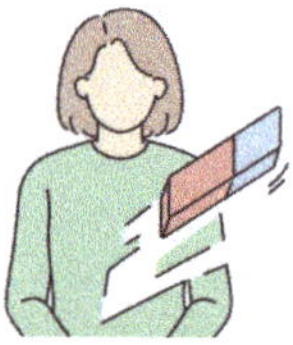

You feel empty or physically numb

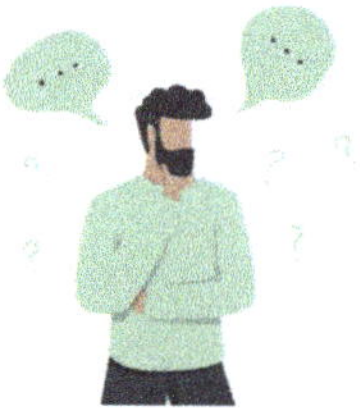

You feel detached from your own thoughts

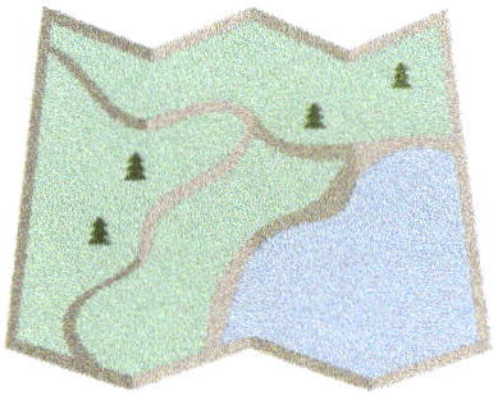

The world seems to be going on without you

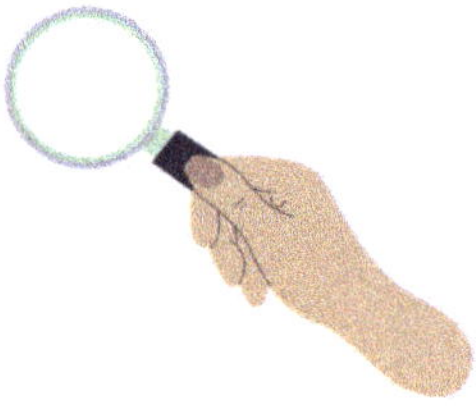

You observe yourself from outside your own body

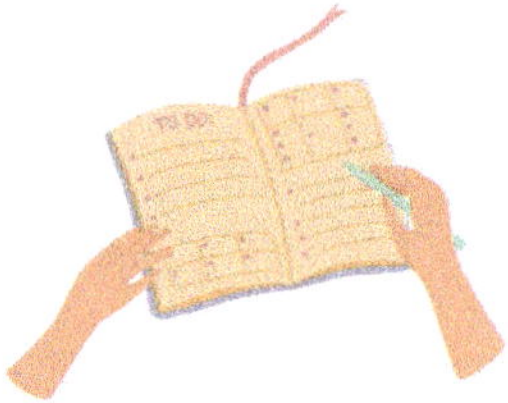

The events of the day or week are hard to recall

"That I shall love always, I argue thee that love is life, and life hath immortality."

Emily Dickinson

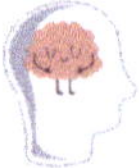

Spend a moment checking in on yourself internally.

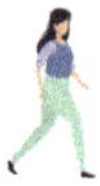

It's important to check in on many different areas of your health because when one of them is affected it often leads to an imbalance and decreased overall well-being.

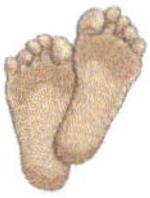

If you do notice a certain area is more often affected you should try to be intentional and take steps to make positive changes.

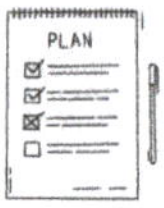

One way you can do this is by creating a daily routine that addresses each area of your health.

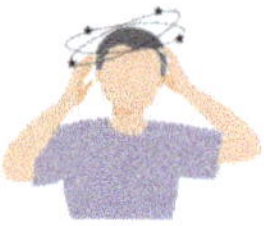

By being intentional and addressing imbalances or problems within your life, you can further shield yourself from mental illness and any other negative mental health affects.

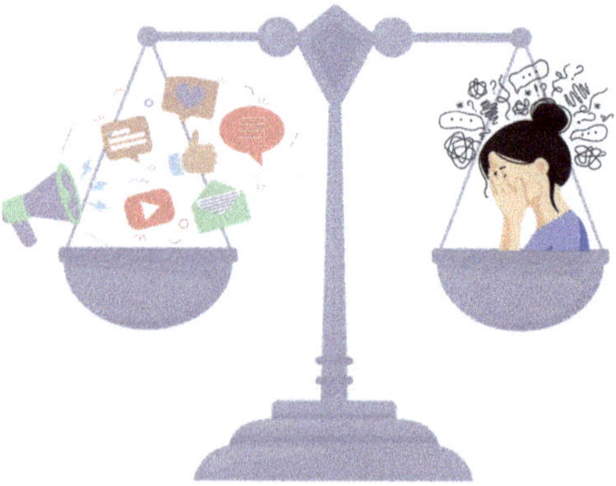

7-11 Breathing

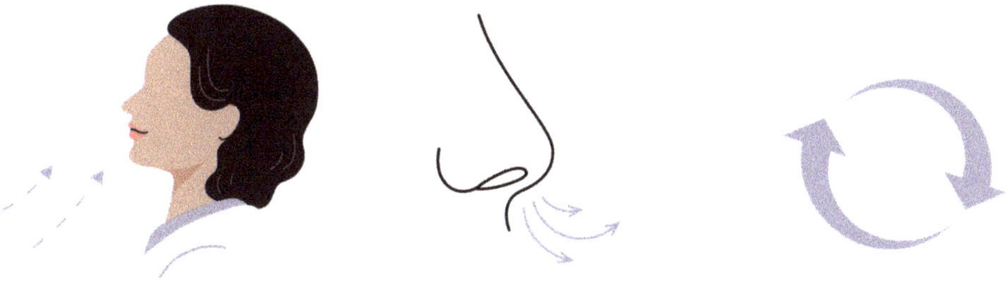

1. Breathe in for 7 seconds
2. Breathe out for 11 seconds
3. Repeat for 10-15 minutes

Take 5-10 minutes to practice your 7-11 breathing in a safe and comfortable environment. During this time, ground yourself then prepare to be vulnerable before you begin to write.

Write for 5 minutes about whatever comes to your mind. Just free write on the next page; no need to judge your thoughts. Just get it out; then breathe through it to lessen the thoughts' power and hold over you.

Take as many more 7-11 breaths as you need before moving on with your day. Practice letting go of your thoughts and resetting. Imagine pushing an internal reset button- roll your shoulders a few times, figure out what you need at this moment; one more 7-11 breath and then move forward!

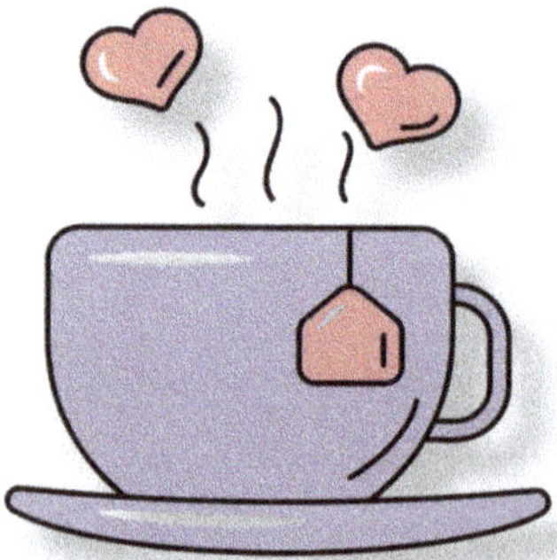

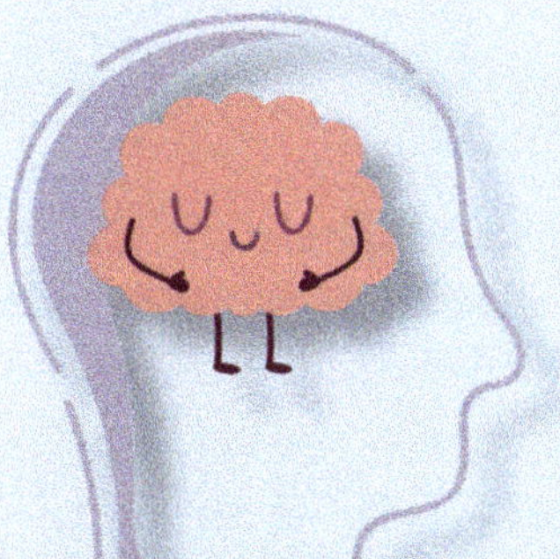

day

23

You're A Rockstar

Shame is an intense feeling of embarrassment, humiliation, or disgrace that arises when a person believes they have failed to meet certain social standards or expectations- what we believe about how we are perceived in the world. It can result from a sense of inadequacy, failure, or wrong-doing, and can be accompanied by feelings of guilt or self-blame. (p.336)

Do You Believe in Magic?

Pretend you have a magic wand and you can change your life into anything you want. What would that look like for you?

Forgive Yourself For...

Not prioritizing yourself

The times you didn't stand up for yourself

Taking breaks

Being hard on yourself

Mistakes you made in the past

Failed relationships

- Forgiveness is an important act of self care.
- We tend to judge ourselves harshly for our mistakes and shortcomings, when we should instead be kind and gracious to ourselves.
- It's important for us to keep our expectations for ourselves realistic.
- One way you can do this is by creating a daily routine that addresses each area of your health.
- One thing to remind yourself is that it's completely normal to make mistakes, this is part of the human experience.

How do you practice self kindness towards yourself?

"How to be happy

Each person deserves a day away in which no problems are confronted, no solutions are searched for."

Maya Angelou

What are you most proud of right now, in this moment?

What are you most proud of right now, in this moment? Write yourself a YOU'RE A ROCKSTAR letter.

day

24

REST

Beliefs are thoughts and feelings that we believe to be true or accept to be true about yourself regardless of evidence or fact. Our beliefs can come from our upbringing, past experiences, social interactions, education, culture, societal norms and relationships. The beliefs that we hold often inform our actions, decision-making, feelings and behaviors that we value impacting the way we think. (p.330)

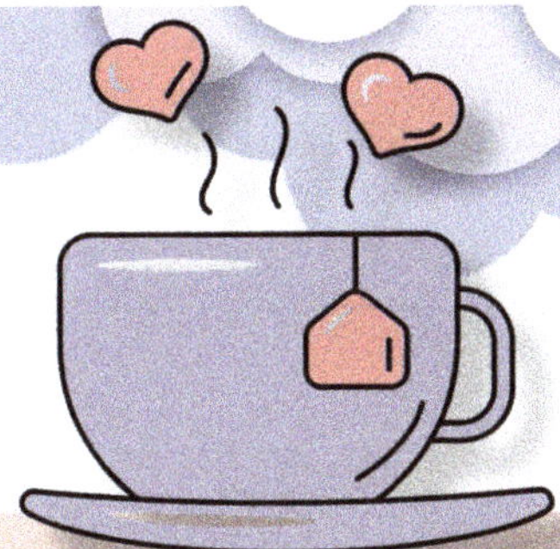

When I take care of myself, I....

I cannot control		I can control
The behavior of others around me	→	My response to other peoples behavior
The future	→	My outlook on life
What others say to me	→	How I choose to let other peoples words affect me
How others treat me	→	The way I treat myself
The beliefs and perceptions of others	→	The way I speak to myself

Spend more time focusing on the things you can control rather than the things you can't!

You cannot always control other's opinions about you, meet others' needs, or fix past mistakes.

However, you can control your attitude, your decisions, and the way you treat others each day.

By focusing on the things you can control and what you can accomplish each day you will be able to reframe negative thoughts about yourself and reduce rumination.

Try making a list of the hings you can control, write below and put it on your mirror!

Limiting Beliefs

Identify areas that you're trying to control, causing you to limit your beliefs. These limiting beliefs are holding you back; you can reframe these thoughts, opening your growth mindset and becoming more productive.

Current limiting belief		Growth mindset reframe
e.g. I'm always giving to people in my life but they're never there for me!	→	e.g. I do not need to stay in toxic relationships, I have the right to be respected.

Current limiting belief

Growth mindset reframe

Butterfly Hug

"The "Butterfly Hug" (BH) is a self-administered Bilateral Stimulation (BLS) method (like the eye movement or tapping) to process traumatic material for an individual or for group work. Desensitization (self-soothing) is a reprocessing byproduct using the BH as BLS." (Artigas & Jarero, 2014)

1. Cross your arms over your chest and point your fingers towards your neck.

2. Slowly move your hands and tap your shoulders like the flapping of butterfly wings - find a speed that feels calming to you.

3. Take slow deep belly breaths and try to clear your mind

4. Do this as many times as you need until you begin to feel more relaxed

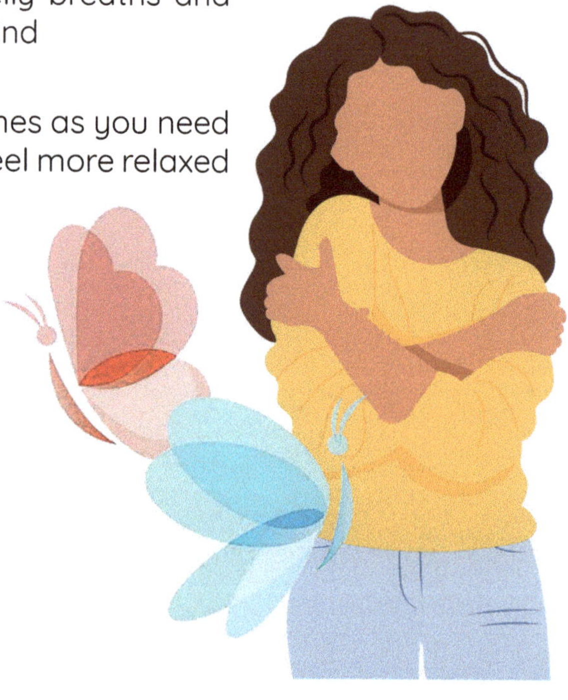

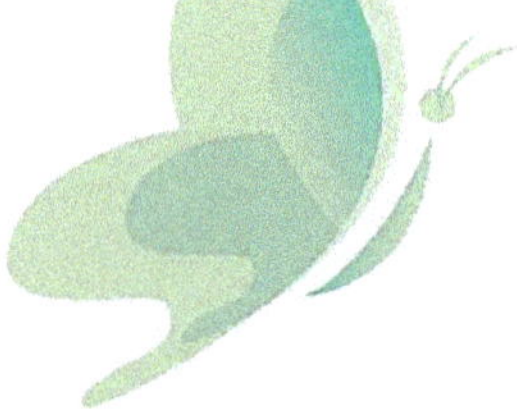

DBT's REST

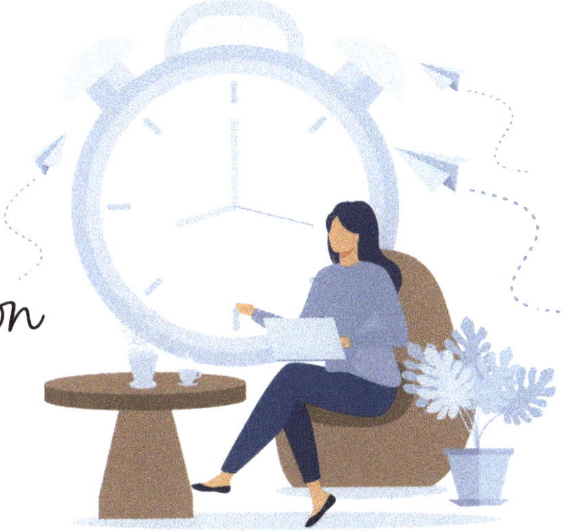

R Relax
E Evaluate
S Set an Intention
T Take Action

What are some ways you can relax?

day 25

Create More Joy

Joy is our level of happiness or satisfaction within our daily lives. This emotion of happiness is often evoked by good well-being and is the result of something positive happening to us. Although we derive joy from successes and good events, we can also create our own joy and happiness through our daily intentions and actions. (p.334)

The Dream Meditation

You Can Do This Anywhere!

1 Find a comfortable place to sit or lie down

2 Take 3 belly breaths before reading each line(use 4X4 deep breathing on p.297)

3 On each deep breath, raise your arms above your head to get a good stretch

The Dream

I have a magic wand.
I can't change the past.
I can control only me.
I can live tomorrow differently.
I use my magic wand and
create a better me!

Tomorrow will be different because...

I believe I can make my DREAM a reality by...

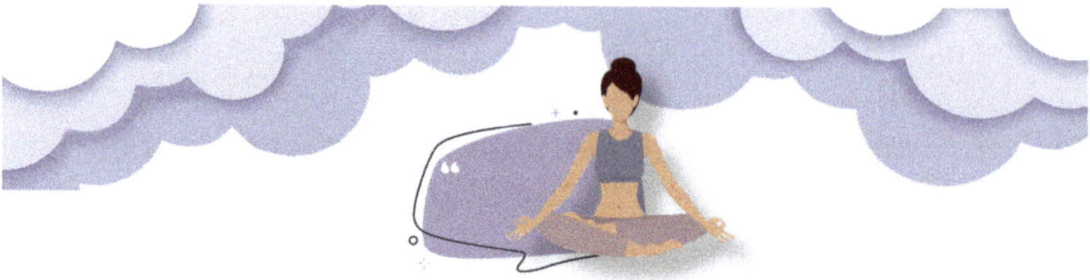

After doing the meditation,
reflect on the following question:

Tomorrow will be different because...

I can make my dream a reality by...

Ways to Become More Present

Take a break
from social media

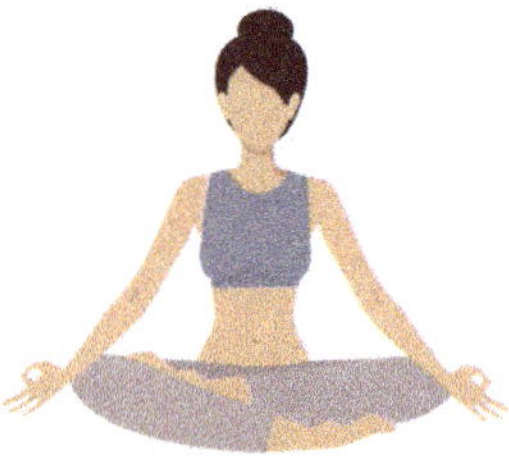

Practice
mindfulness

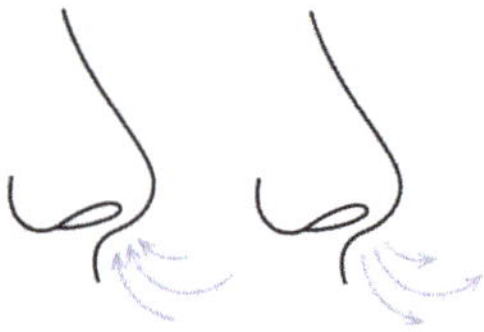

Focus on
your breathing

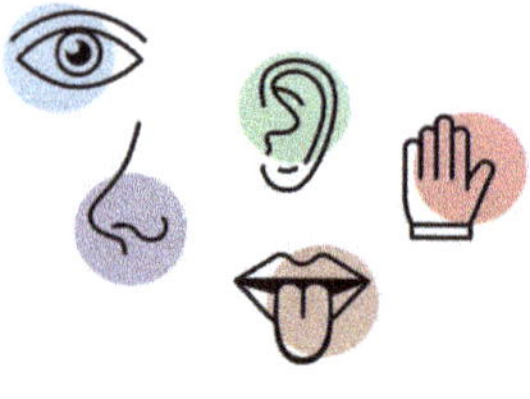

Connect with
your 5 senses

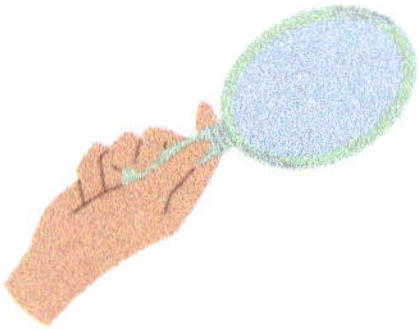

Reflect on
each day

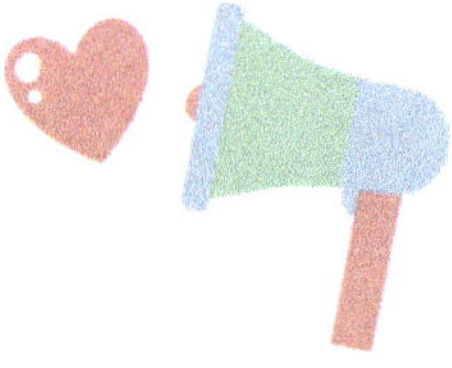

Think about
who/what you
are grateful for

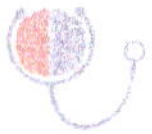

As our minds spiral through anxious thoughts, we can experience worry, panic, and fear.

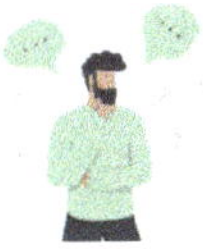

The good news is that there are ways that we can escape anxious thoughts and return to the present moment in order to calm down quickly.

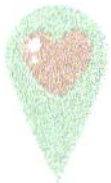

Using these techniques, we can become more aware of our current experiences and engage more with life in the present moment.

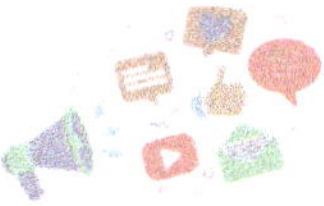

Try limiting your social media usage instead of mindlessly scrolling to cope with your emotions. This may assist you in recognizing and acknowledging your emotions.

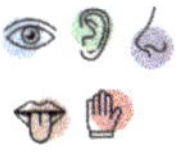

In addition, try engaging your five senses. Practicing this will help you ground yourself, connect with your environment, and eliminate panic.

Creating More Joy

Ask yourself and write your answers below

WHAT activities bring me joy?

Creating More Joy

Ask yourself and write your answers below

WHEN do I feel confident?

Creating More Joy

Ask yourself and write your answers below

AM I letting go of my mistakes made?

Creating More Joy

Ask yourself and write your answers below

WHAT makes me unique?

Creating More Joy

Ask yourself and write your answers below

WHAT makes me feel most alive?

Tomorrow will be different because...

What can you do to get back to YOU?

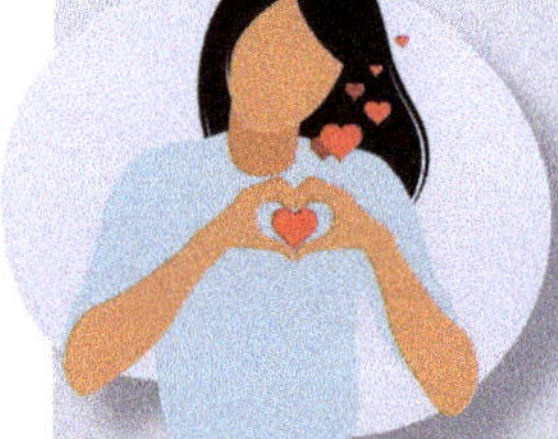

I believe I can make my dream a reality by...

day 26

R.A.I.N

Mindfulness is a practice that involves being fully present and engaged in the present moment, without judgment or distraction. It involves paying attention to your thoughts, feelings, and bodily sensations, and observing them with curiosity and openness. Mindfulness can be practiced through a variety of techniques, such as meditation, breathing exercises, or simply paying attention to your surroundings. (p.334)

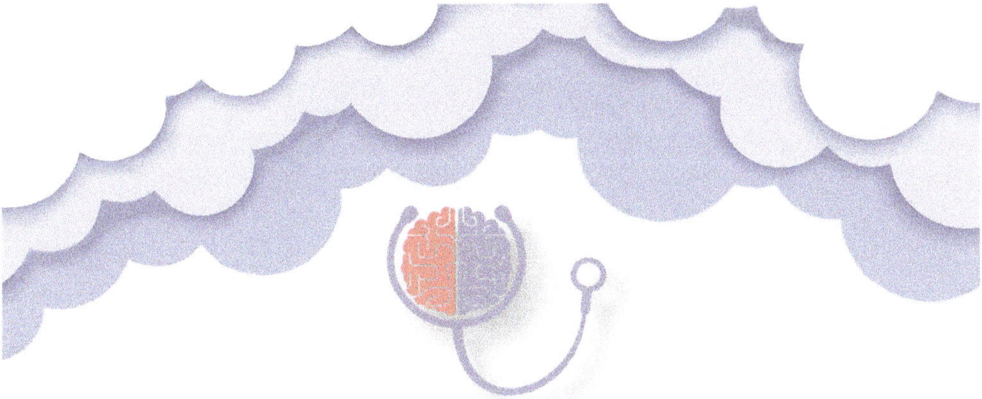

We can find ways to cope through asking for help as well as seeking out support

Where can I get support if I need it?

How will I ask for support if I need it?

What do I need to refuel my spirit?

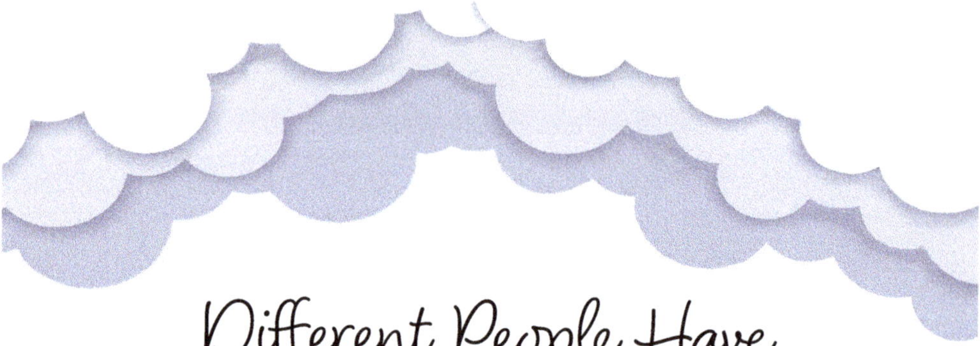

Different People Have Different Needs

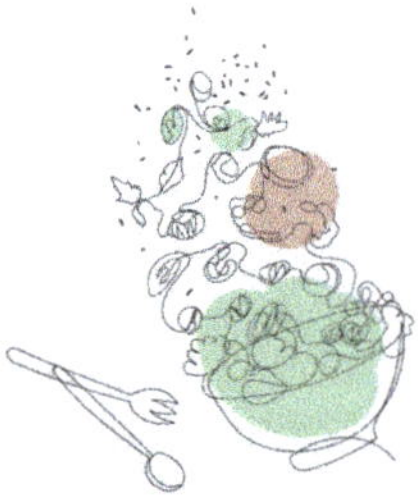

- Lots of exercise
- Clean eating
- No social media

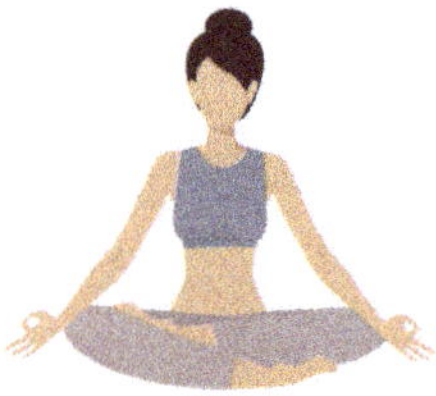

- Meditation
- Creating art
- Indoor plants

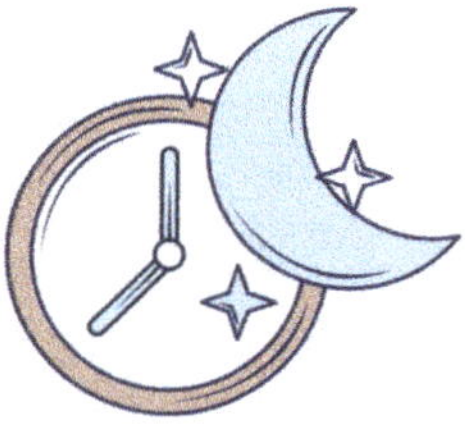

- Lots of sleep
- Reading
- Playing sports

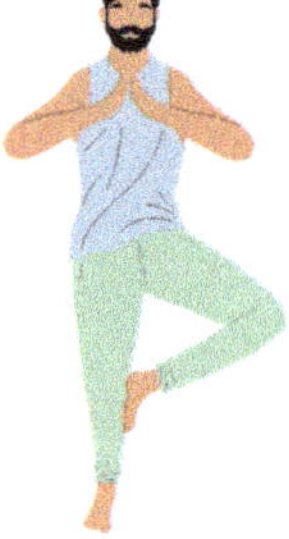

- Yoga
- Alone time
- Journaling

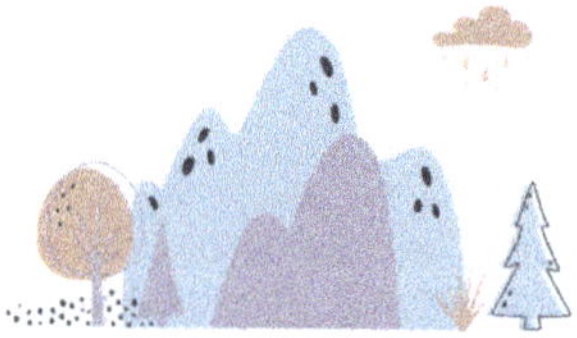

- Time in nature
- Traveling
- Positive content

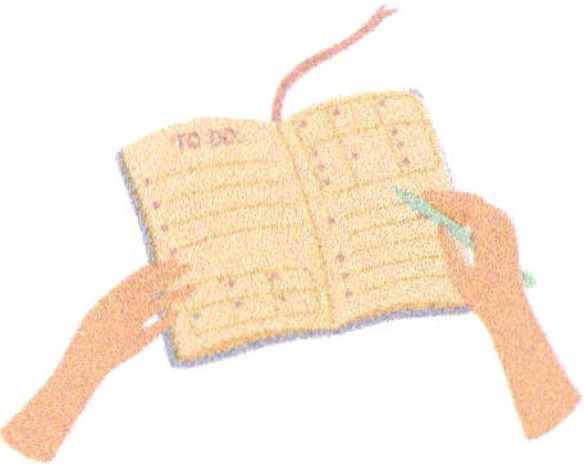

- To-do lists
- Social time
- Therapy

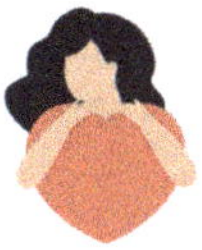

It is important for us to recognize that we are all different and require separate routines and needs.

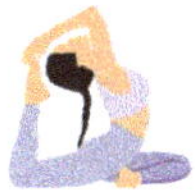

Some people may take care of themselves by eating lots of leafy greens, exercising intensely, and staying off social media, while others may prefer to meditate, paint, and take care of indoor plants.

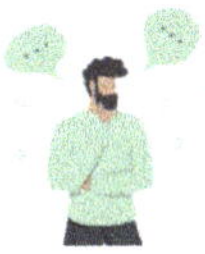

Listening to our bodies and minds is one of the most important things we can do to boost our spirit, mood, and emotions.

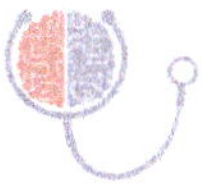

Maintaining healthy routines and activities that bring us joy helps us cope with stress and negative mental health.

Is there anything you couldn't live without in your routine? Write your answer to this below.

Phone-Less Creative Activities

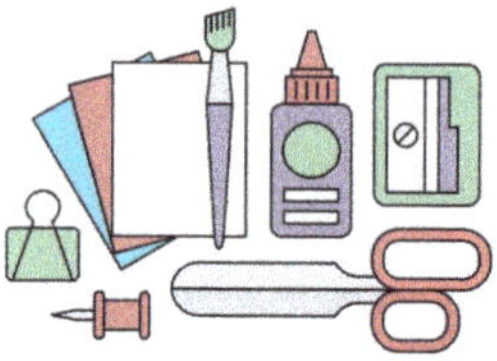

Crafts

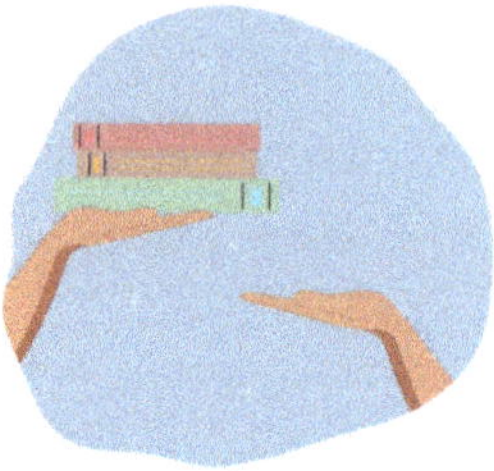

Reading

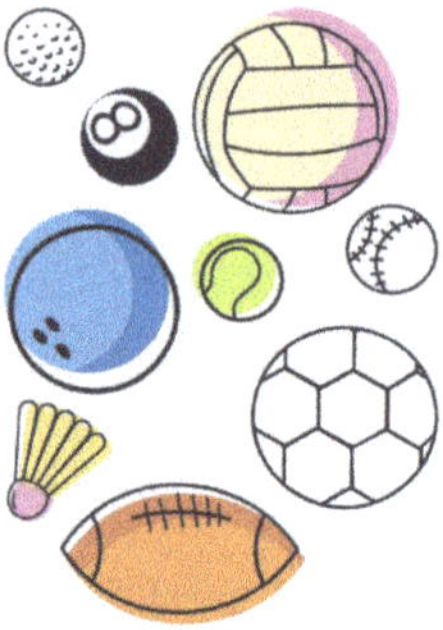

Playing sports

Painting

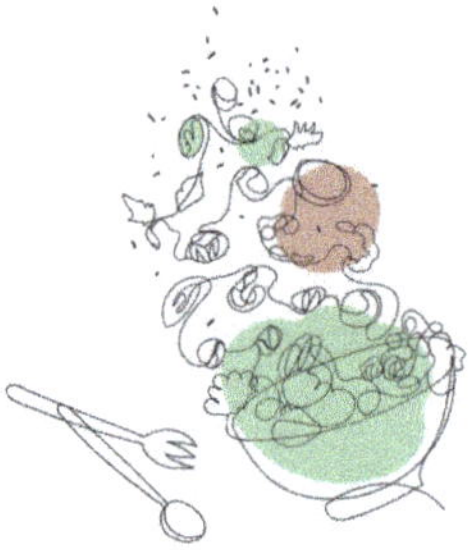

Cooking

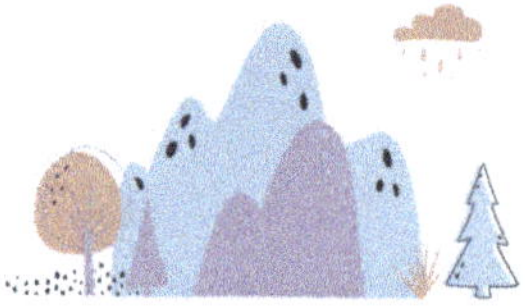

Going for a nature walk

Listening to music

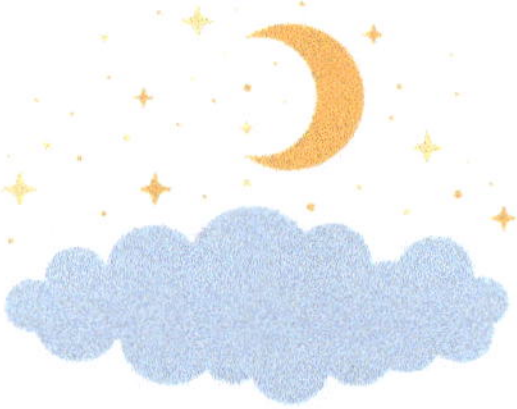

Napping

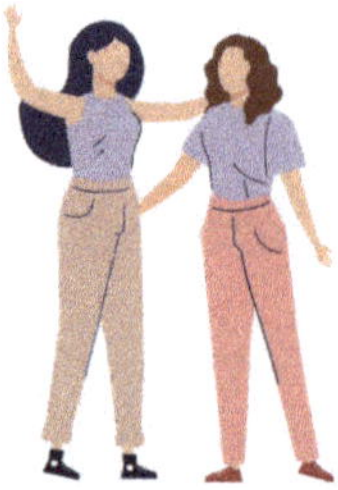

Socializing

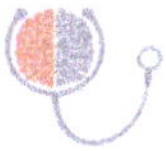

Creativity can benefit our mind in many ways!

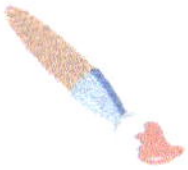

Creative outlets such as drawing, painting, and designing allow us to release stress, which can reduce fatigue, exhaustion, and burnout.

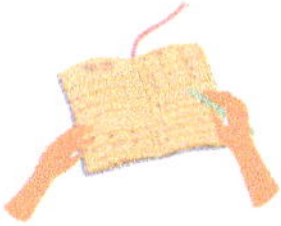

Activities that inspire creativity also allow us to express how we feel, which can also be very therapeutic.

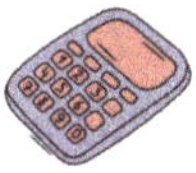

Additionally, with practice, you can develop a great deal of skill and pride in what you're doing, instilling a sense of confidence in yourself.

Schedule a creative activity once a week and see how it benefits you! List your top 3 things below:

Doodle for 5 minutes

Doodling makes us smile... how did doodling make you feel?

RAIN MINDFULNESS

Bringing mindful awareness to emotional distress

R Recognize what is happening in this moment

A Allow life to be as it is

I Investigate with kind-ness/interest/care

N Nurture the thought that you are not defined by an uncomfortable feeling/ emotion

Color Me

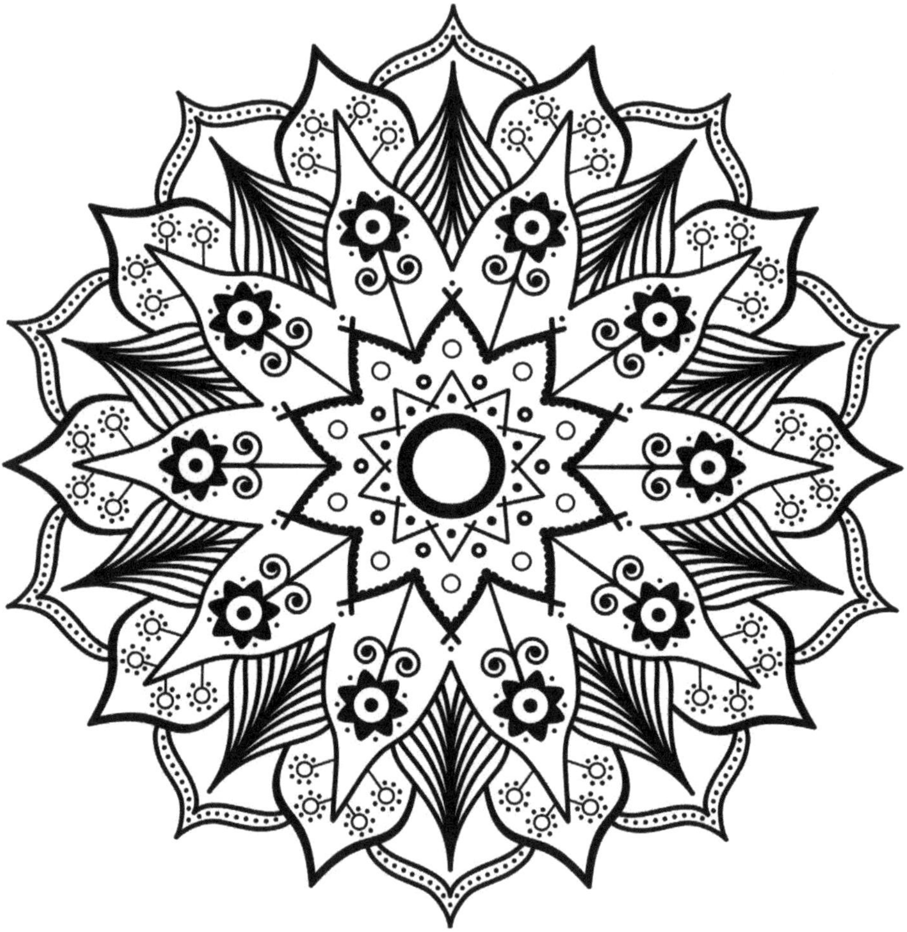

Color Me

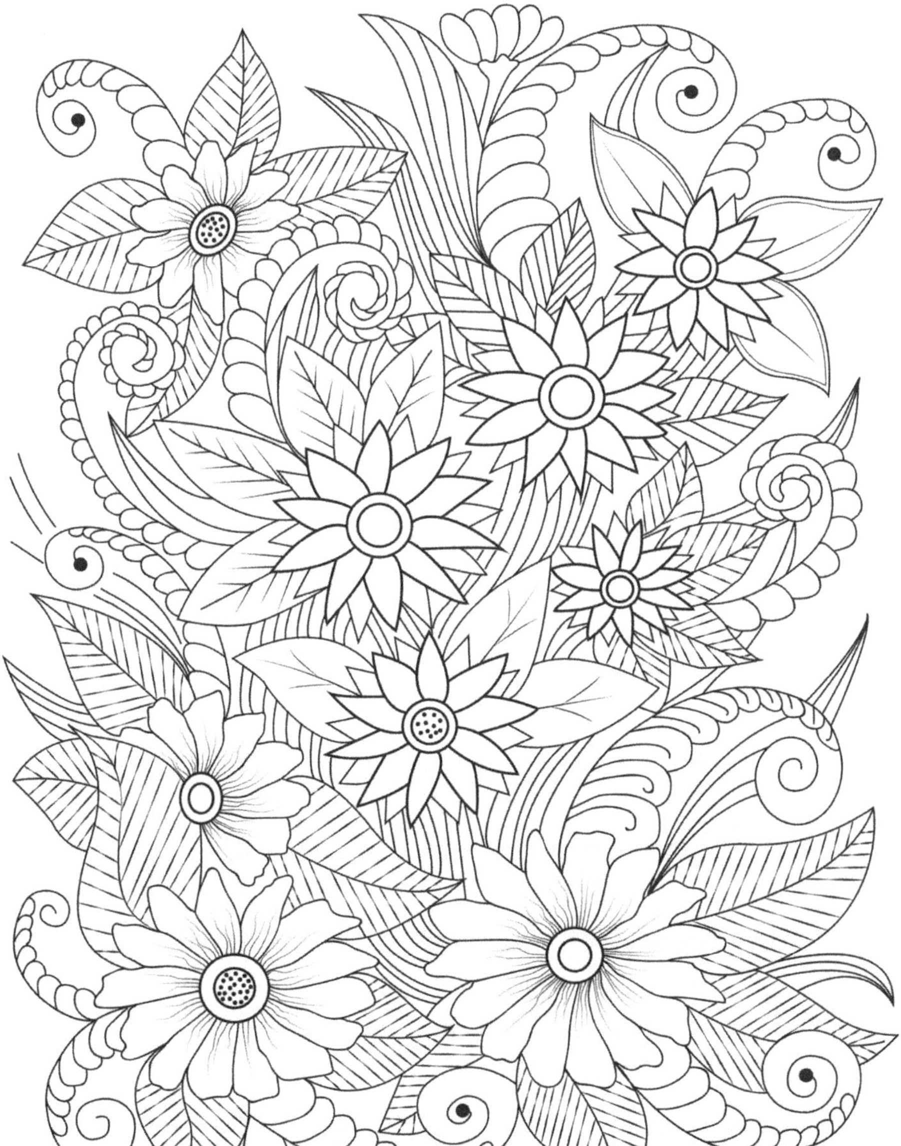

day 27

Get Happy

Happiness is a positive emotional state characterized by feelings of contentment, satisfaction, and pleasure. It is often associated with joy, fulfillment, and a sense of well-being. Happiness can be experienced in response to various stimuli, such as achieving a goal, spending time with loved ones, engaging in activities we enjoy, or simply appreciating the beauty of the world around us. (p.334)

I know I'm happy when I...

Ways to Show Yourself Compassion

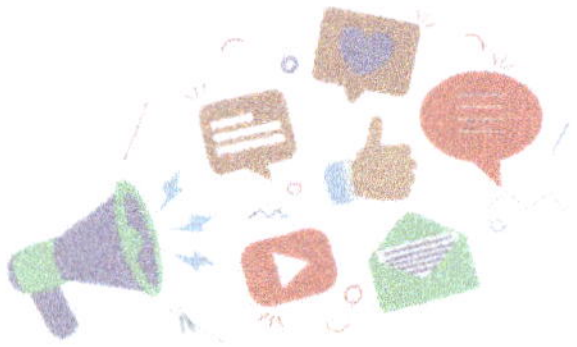

Speak to yourself as you would to a friend

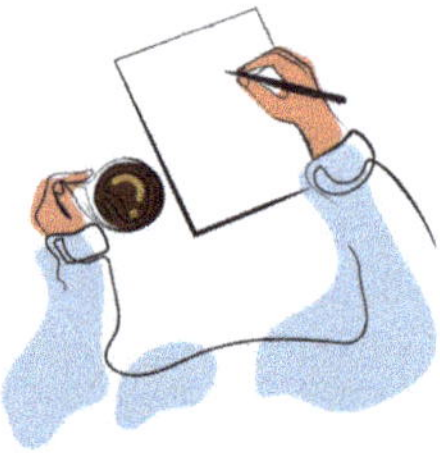

Write yourself an encouraging letter

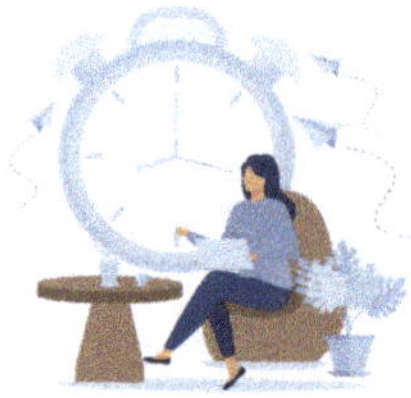

Give your mind and body a rest

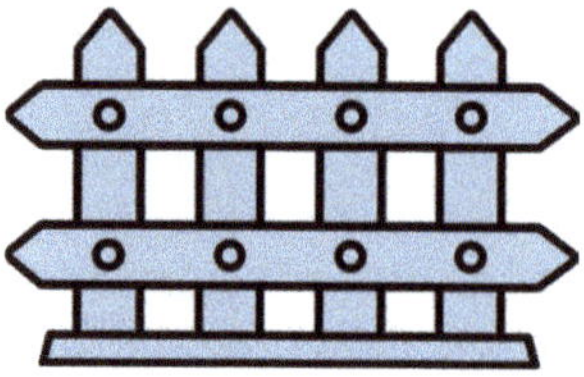

Set healthy boundaries with others

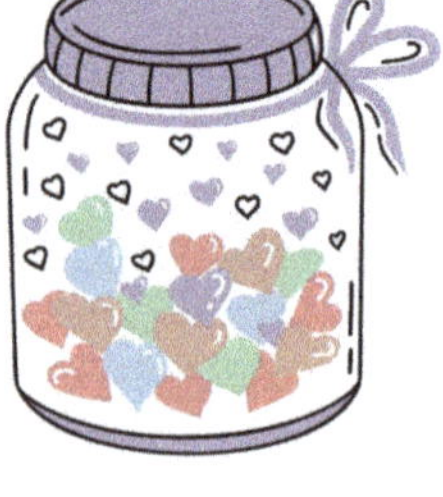

Don't push yourself too hard

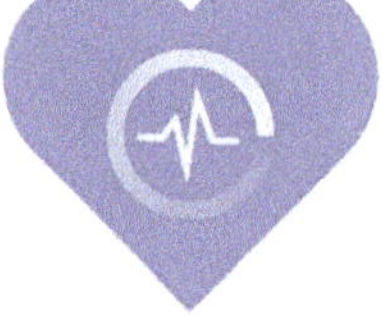

Give yourself a treat that makes you smile

To express self-compassion, consider:
- Self-compassionate phrases
- Treating yourself as you would treat a friend
- Practicing mindfulness, and
- Granting yourself permission to be human

Recognizing that imperfection is a universal human experience is key to offering yourself forgiveness.

Also, it's important to make time for activities that bring you happiness.

By adopting these practices, you can enhance your well-being and mental health. What are you willing to try?

Make a list below of the things you are willing to try:

Gratitude Jar

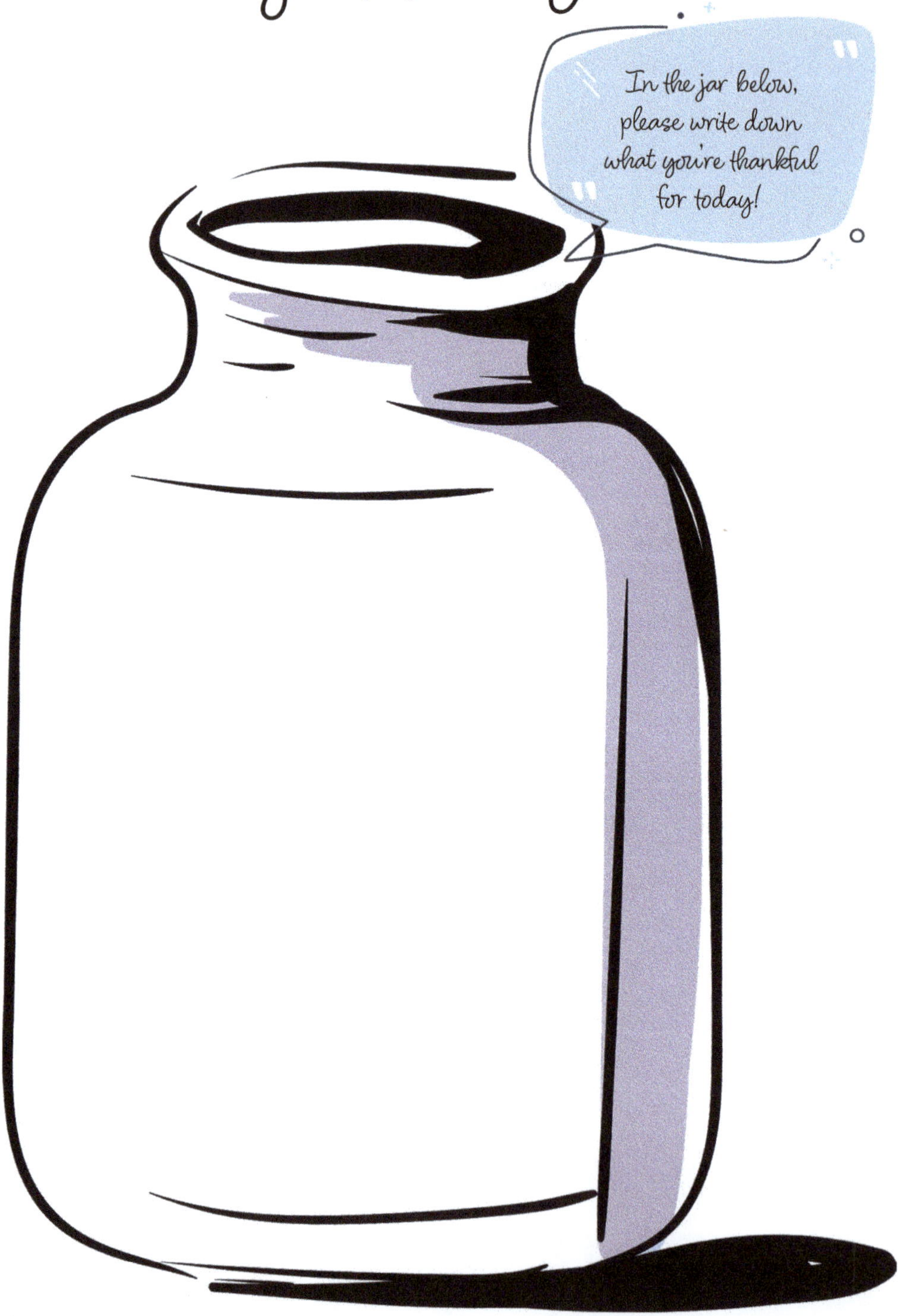

One Gratitude For The Day

Sunday

Monday

Tuesday

Wednesday

Thursday

Friday

Saturday

Self-Love Reminders

You are allowed to feel your feelings

Your needs are valid

You are stronger than you think

Your boundaries matter

You are worthy of love

You are important and you matter

Mental illness does not define you

It's okay to have bad days

Friendly reminders that you are doing amazing!

Don't forget that you are valued, loved and appreciated by so many.

You can only do your best, and that is enough.

Remember to treat yourself kindly and to allow yourself breaks when necessary.

You are never a burden and the space you take up is important!

How will you take up space today?

Happiness Boosters

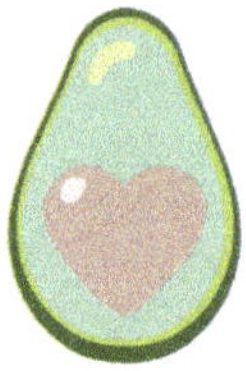

Eat healthy foods

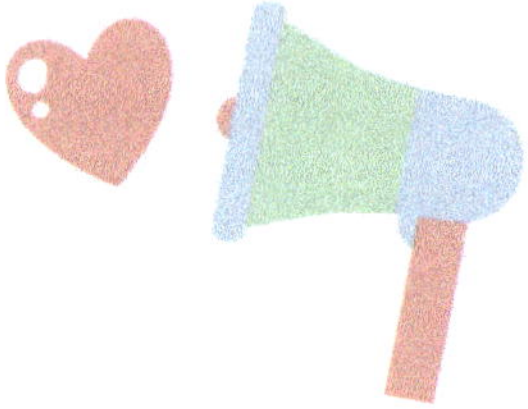

Express kindness

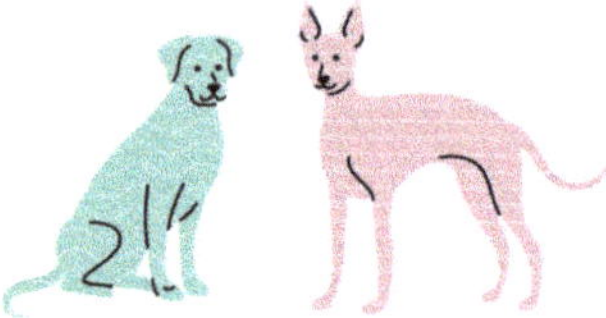

Play with your pets

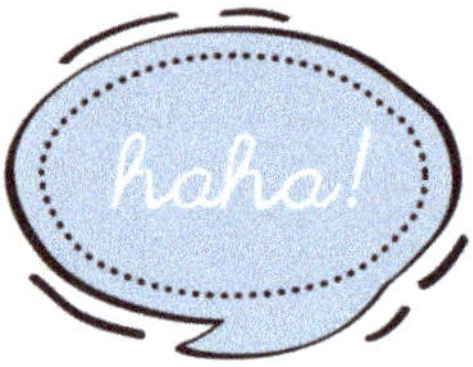

Watch a funny video

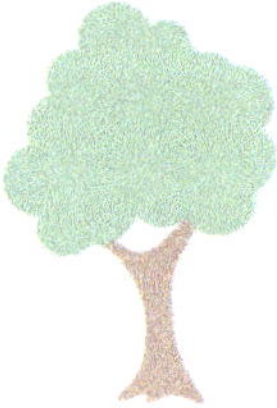

Take a walk outdoors

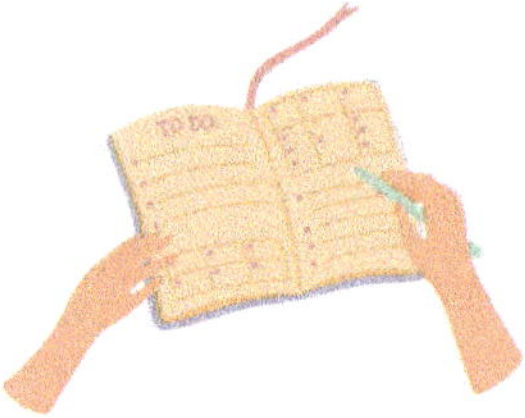

Complete a task

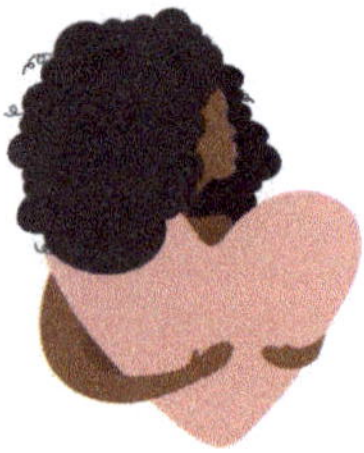

Hug someone

Get direct sunlight

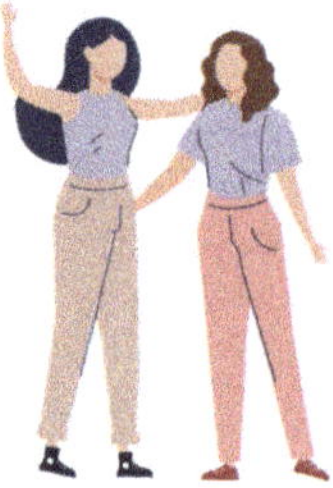

Spend time with friends

Did you know there are many simple ways you can boost your happiness?

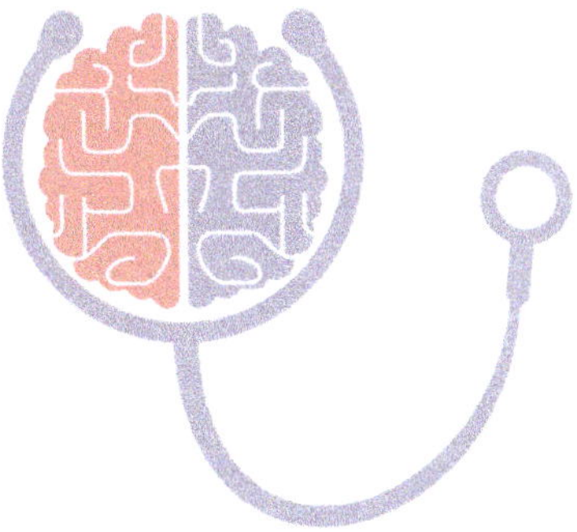

Happy brain chemicals such as dopamine, oxytocin, serotonin, and endorphins can be produced naturally through activities such as exercising, laughing, social connection, expressing kindness and more.

These hormones help to ease depression and anxiety while promoting happiness and pleasure.

Ways to active them:

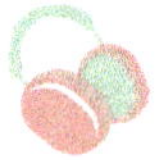

Dopamine: Complete a task, listen to music, and try something new.

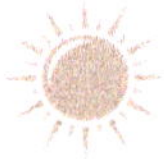

Serotonin: Get sunlight, exercise, meditate, and maintain a healthy diet.

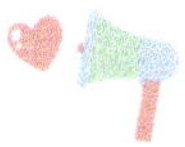

Oxytocin: Get/give a massage, spend time with friends, show affection, and do something kind.

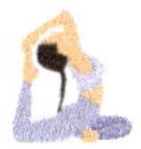

Endorphins: Exercise regularly, practice yoga or meditation, create art and laugh.

List of Pleasurable Distractions

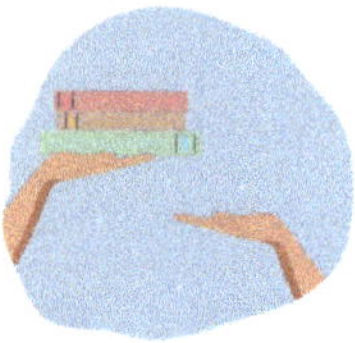
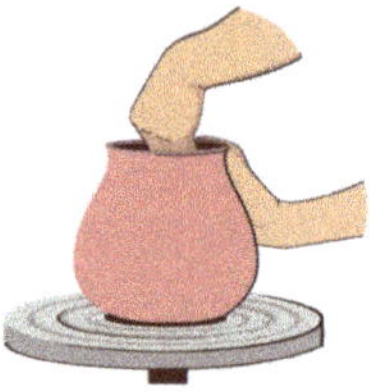
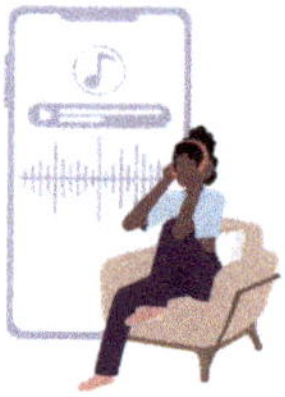
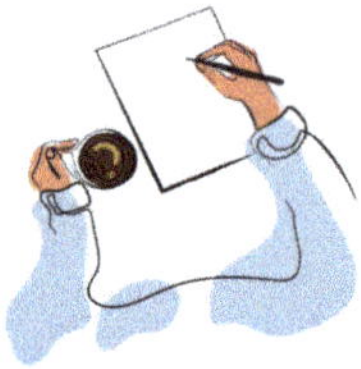

Place checkmarks next to the activities that you enjoy

- [ ] Exercising
- [ ] Talking to friends
- [ ] Taking a hot bath
- [ ] Aromatherapy
- [ ] Reading a book
- [ ] Watching a movie
- [ ] Playing sports
- [ ] Singing & dancing
- [ ] Taking an online class
- [ ] Joining a club
- [ ] Journaling
- [ ] Painting your nails
- [ ] Meditation
- [ ] Taking a nap
- [ ] Cooking and baking
- [ ] Solving a puzzle
- [ ] Riding a bike
- [ ] Cleaning
- [ ] Listening to music
- [ ] Practicing yoga
- [ ] Calling a friend
- [ ] Coloring
- [ ] Decluttering your room
- [ ] Learning something new

Make a list of all the beautiful things you see right now, in this moment:

1

2

3

4

5

6

7

8

9

10

day 28

Be Your Own Superhero

Character Traits are our unique individual qualities or attributes that make us who we are. Many of us have unique qualities that impact our personality and how we relate to others. It's important to identify your unique thoughts and behaviors as well as how they can be your "superpowers" within your life. (p.331)

Daily Reflection

YAY Me- I was great today when:

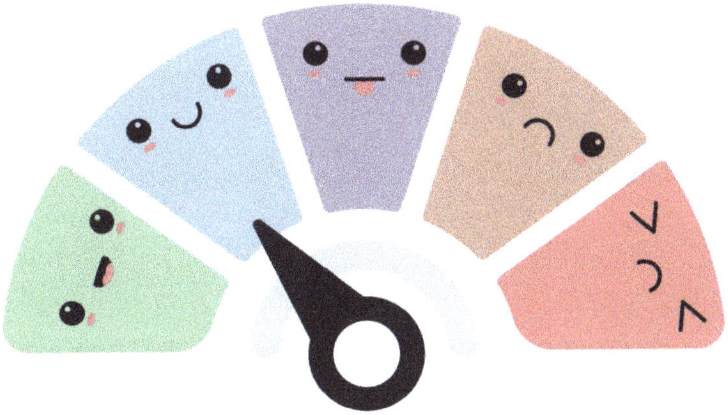

Today's act of kindness:

Reason for my rating:

Something new I learned today:

The Many Types of STRONG

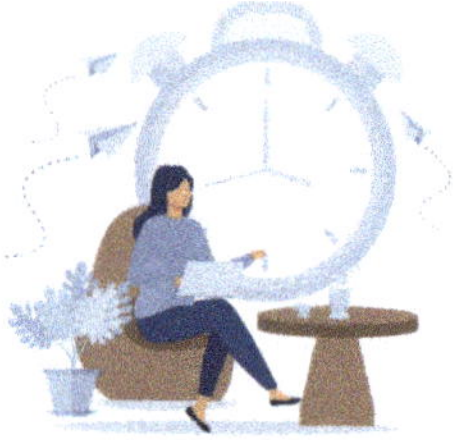

Choosing to rest instead of pushing yourself

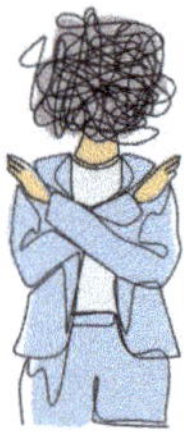

Facing painful thoughts and moving forward

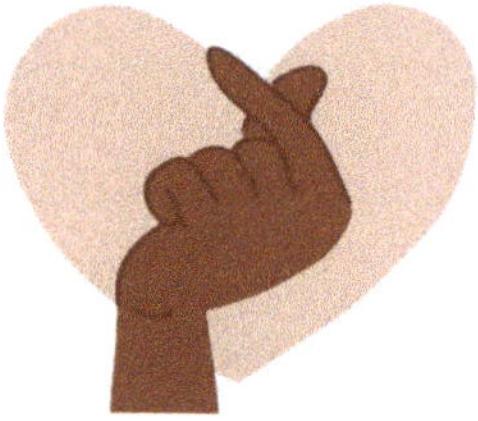

Truly seeing and validating yourself

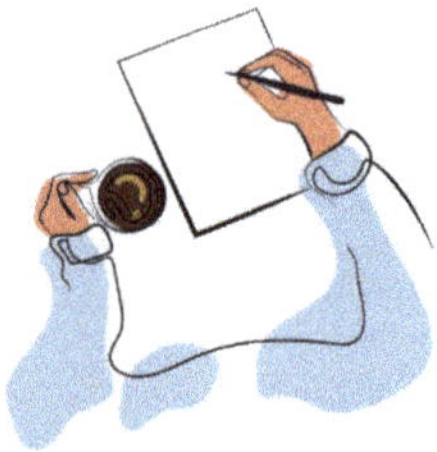

Choosing healing even when it's messy

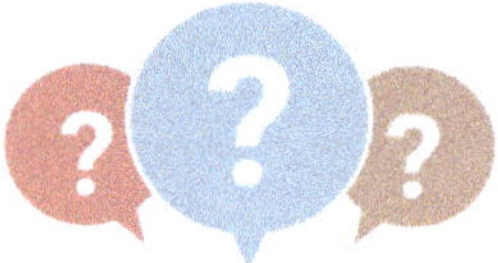

Believing even when things don't make sense

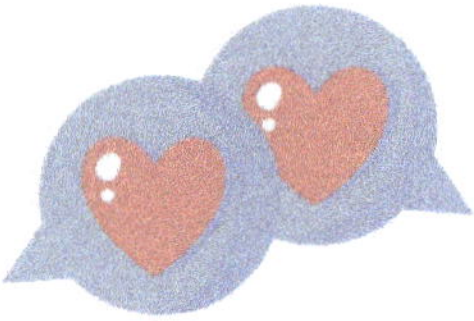

Telling someone about the way you're feeling

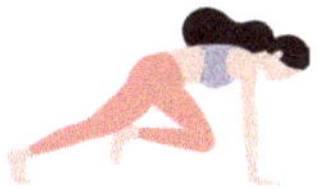

Being strong is more than being physically tough or making hard decisions.

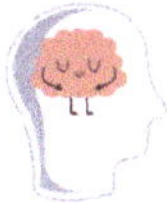

It's also making decisions that are beneficial for your mental health and committing to becoming the best version of yourself.

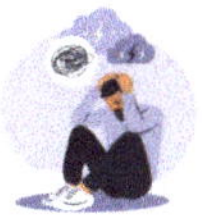

It's not an easy decision to let others know we are struggling, to seek help, to rest when we are expected to keep pushing, or begin healing!

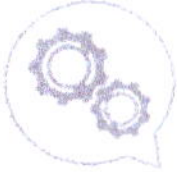

If it was easy we'd all be doing these things.

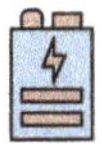

Don't forget how much strength it takes you to advocate and invest in yourself daily.

Create an intention to make this happen today; write it here:

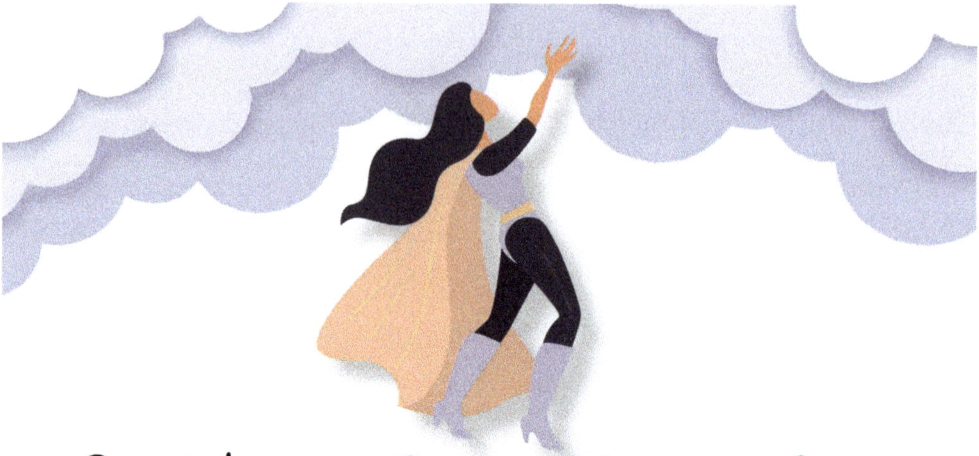

Be Your Own Superhero

MANIFEST YOUR POWER

My Super Power is ______________________________

I am a Super Hero!

I can summon my super power by...

____!

Creating Your Superhero's Character Traits

Make a list of positive traits (honesty, empathetic, loving, etc) that you want to cultivate in yourself.

Identify 5 **YAY ME** Moments

that you've had!

1

2

3

4

5

Why do you feel that they were personal wins for you?

Having a "RUFF" day?

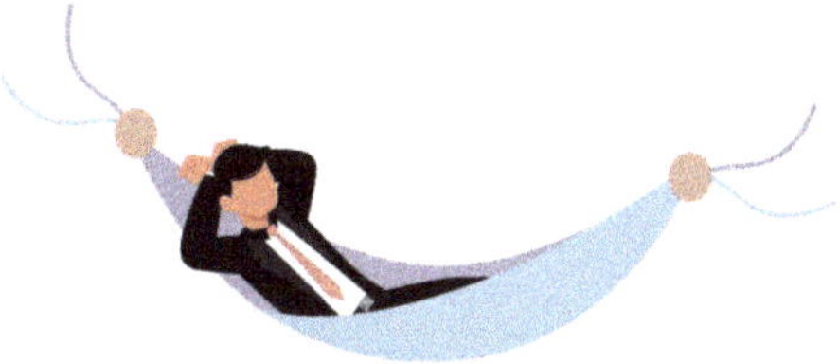

Rest

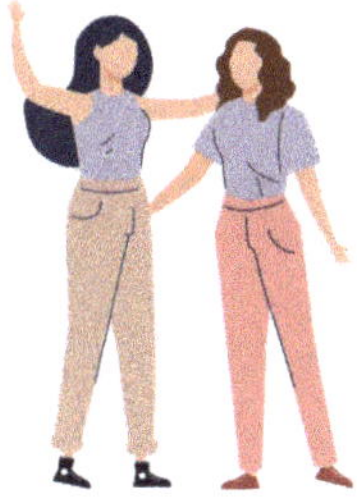

Unplug

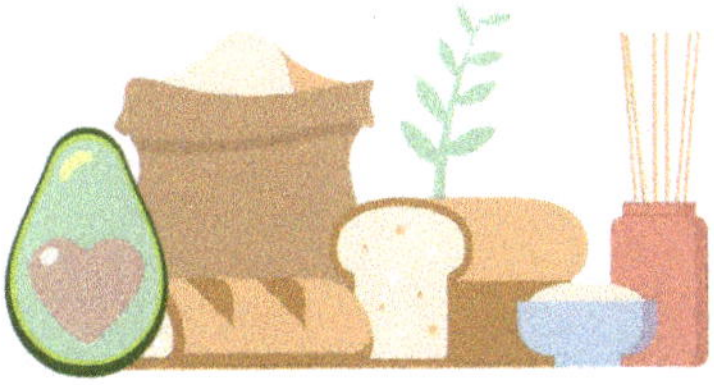

Food

Fun

day 29

Take a Breath

Character Traits are our unique individual qualities or attributes that make us who we are. Many of us have unique qualities that impact our personality and how we relate to others. It's important to identify your unique thoughts and behaviors as well as how they can be your "superpowers" within your life. (p.331)

Having a "RUFF" day?

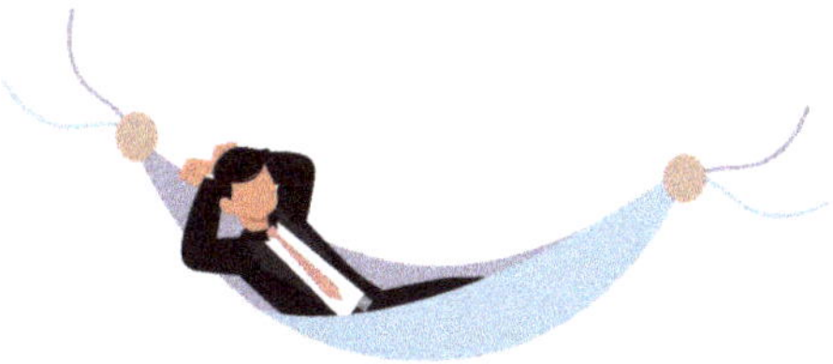

Rest

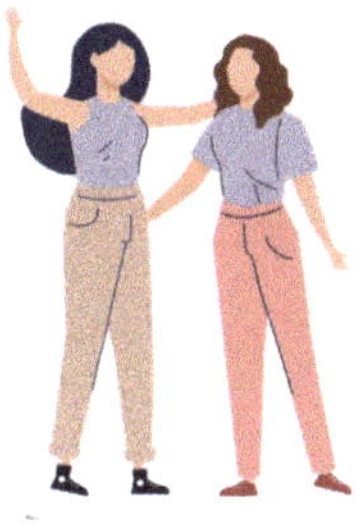

Unplug

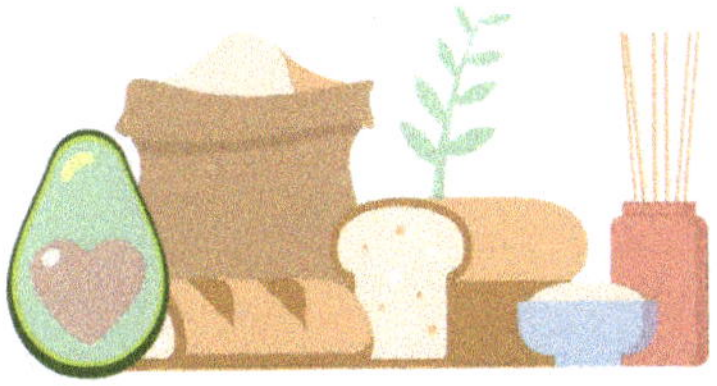

Food

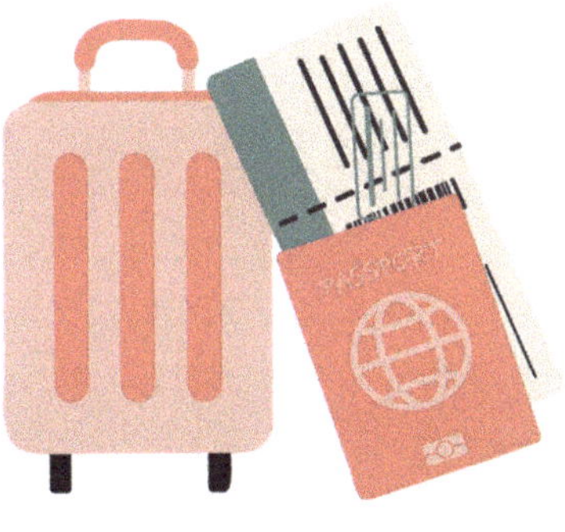

Fun

day 29

Take a Breath

Character Traits are our unique individual qualities or attributes that make us who we are. Many of us have unique qualities that impact our personality and how we relate to others. It's important to identify your unique thoughts and behaviors as well as how they can be your "superpowers" within your life. (p.331)

Things You Don't Need To Justify

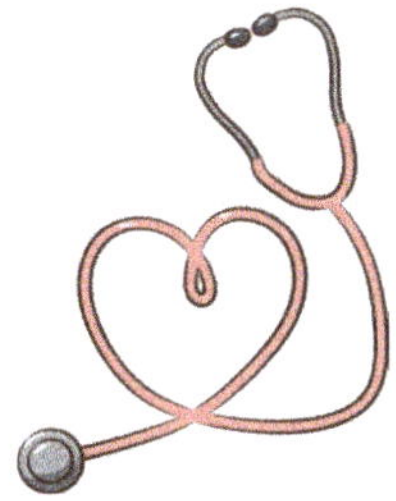

Who you love or why you love them

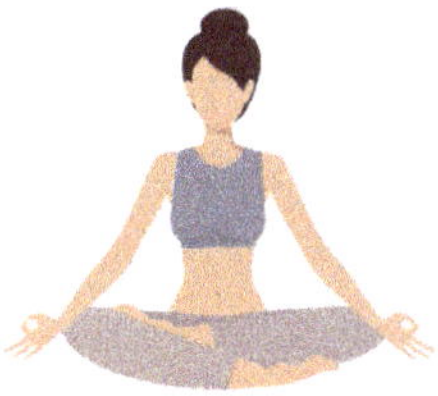

The way you spend your free time

When or how often you take breaks

Ending toxic relationships

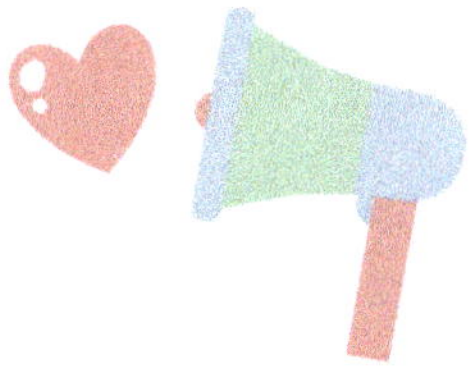

Asking for your needs to be met

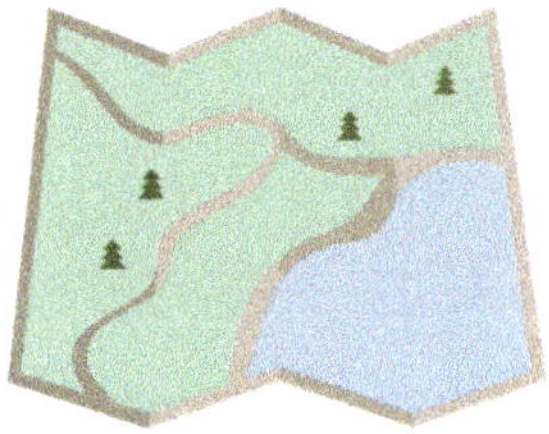

Changing your direction in life

Tips for Moving On

After Making A Mistake

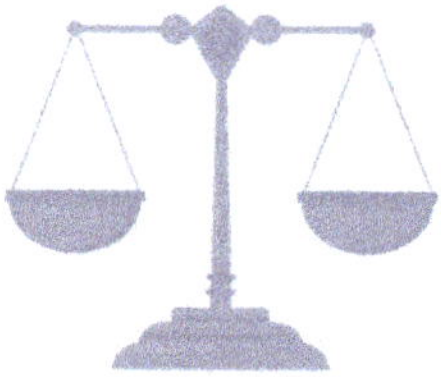

Be honest with yourself and others

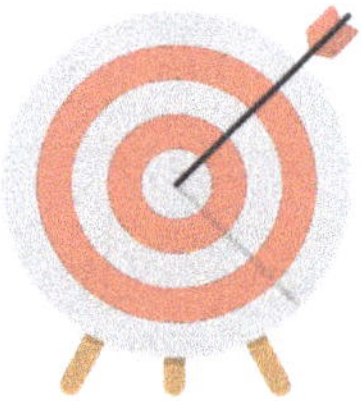

Take responsibility for what you did

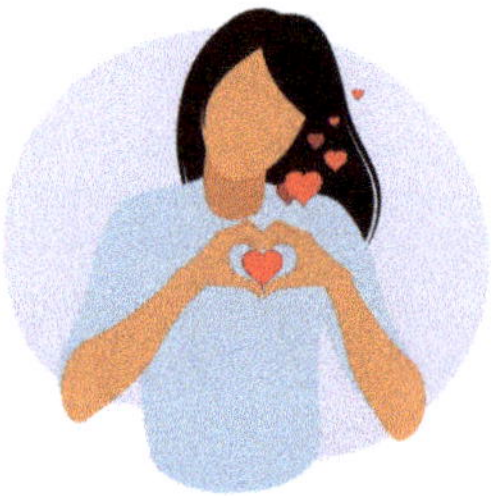

Make amends if you hurt someone

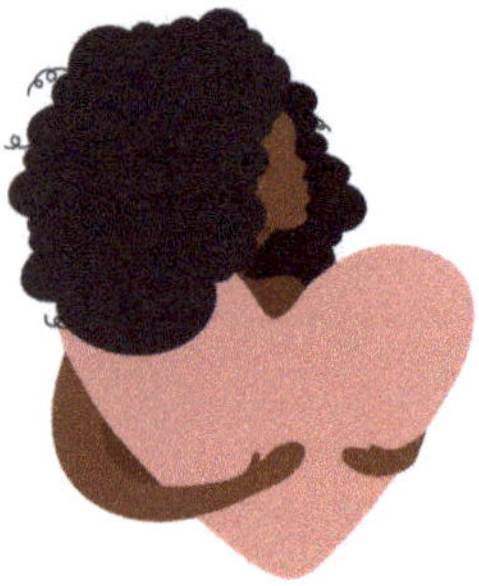

Forgive yourself and move forward

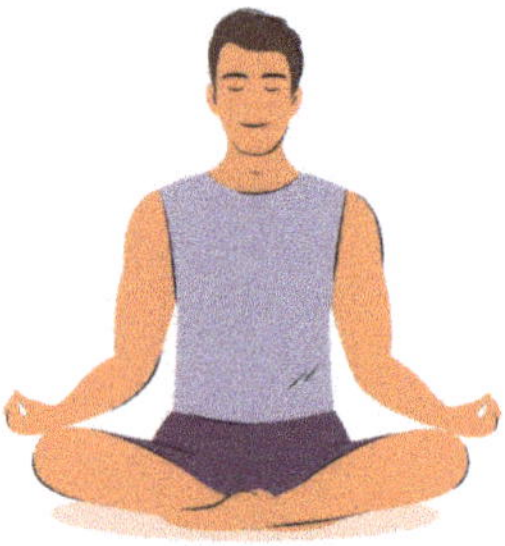

Breathe, regroup, and try again

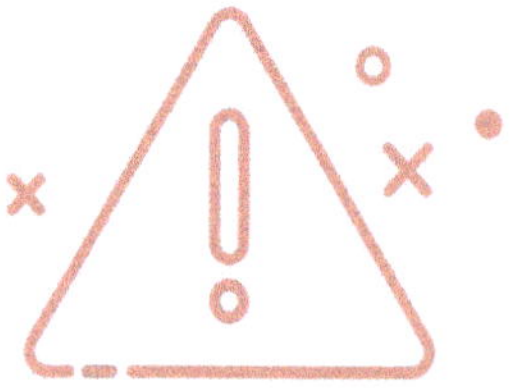

Remember that humans make mistakes

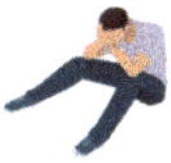

Stuck ruminating on a past mistake? These tips are for you!

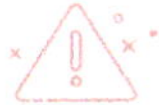

Often, after making a mistake, we judge ourselves very harshly and are very critical of ourselves.

Althoughit'simportanttoapologizetoothersandown uptoourmistakes,weshouldn'tdwellonthemforever.

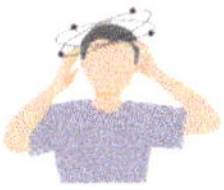

When we ruminate over past mistakes, we only further decrease our mood, heightening anxiety and dissatisfaction with oneself.

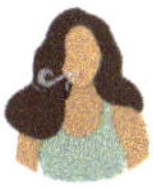

Whenever you make a mistake, it's helpful to focus on your breathing (pg.255), to remind yourself that mistakes are normal, and to forgive yourself.

What do you need to forgive yourself for right now?

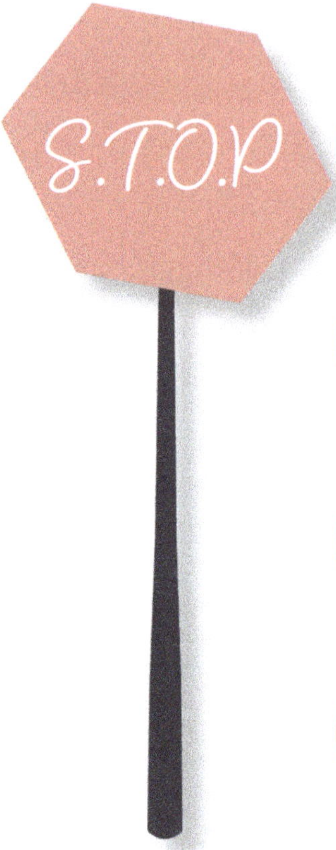

1. Stop
2. Take a breath
3. Observe
4. Proceed

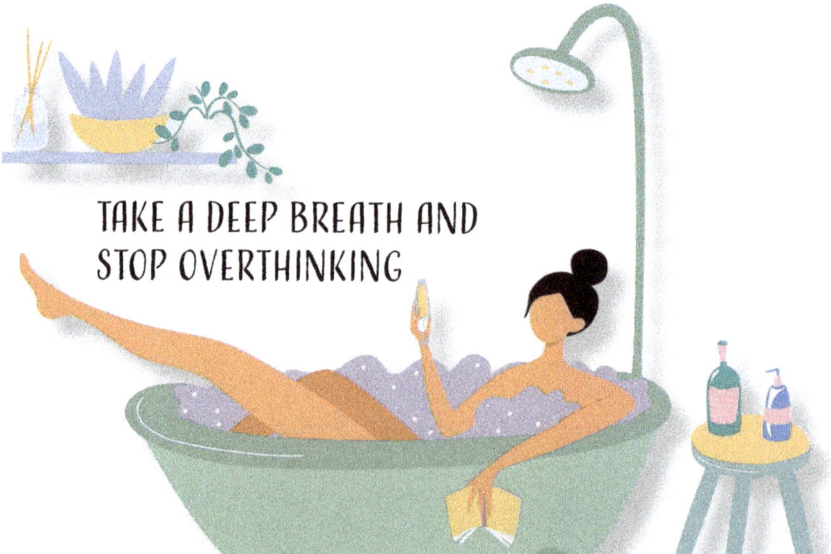

How can you be self compassionate next time you make a mistake?

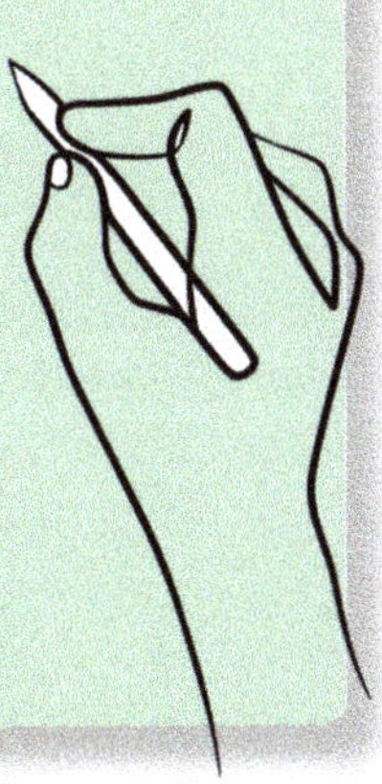

What are you going to do to take care of yourself when mistakes happen?

P.E.A.C.E

1. Pause 
2. Exhale 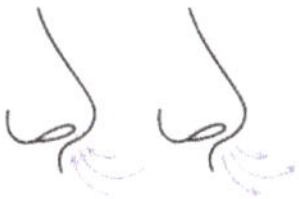
3. Acknowledge 
4. Choose skill 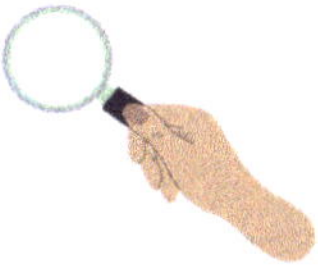
5. Engage skill 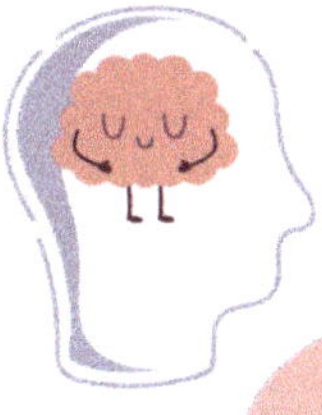

When I do hard things I feel...

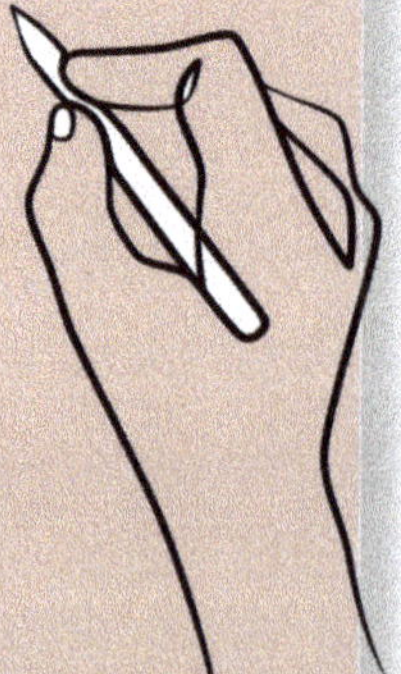

10 Benefits of Deep Breathing

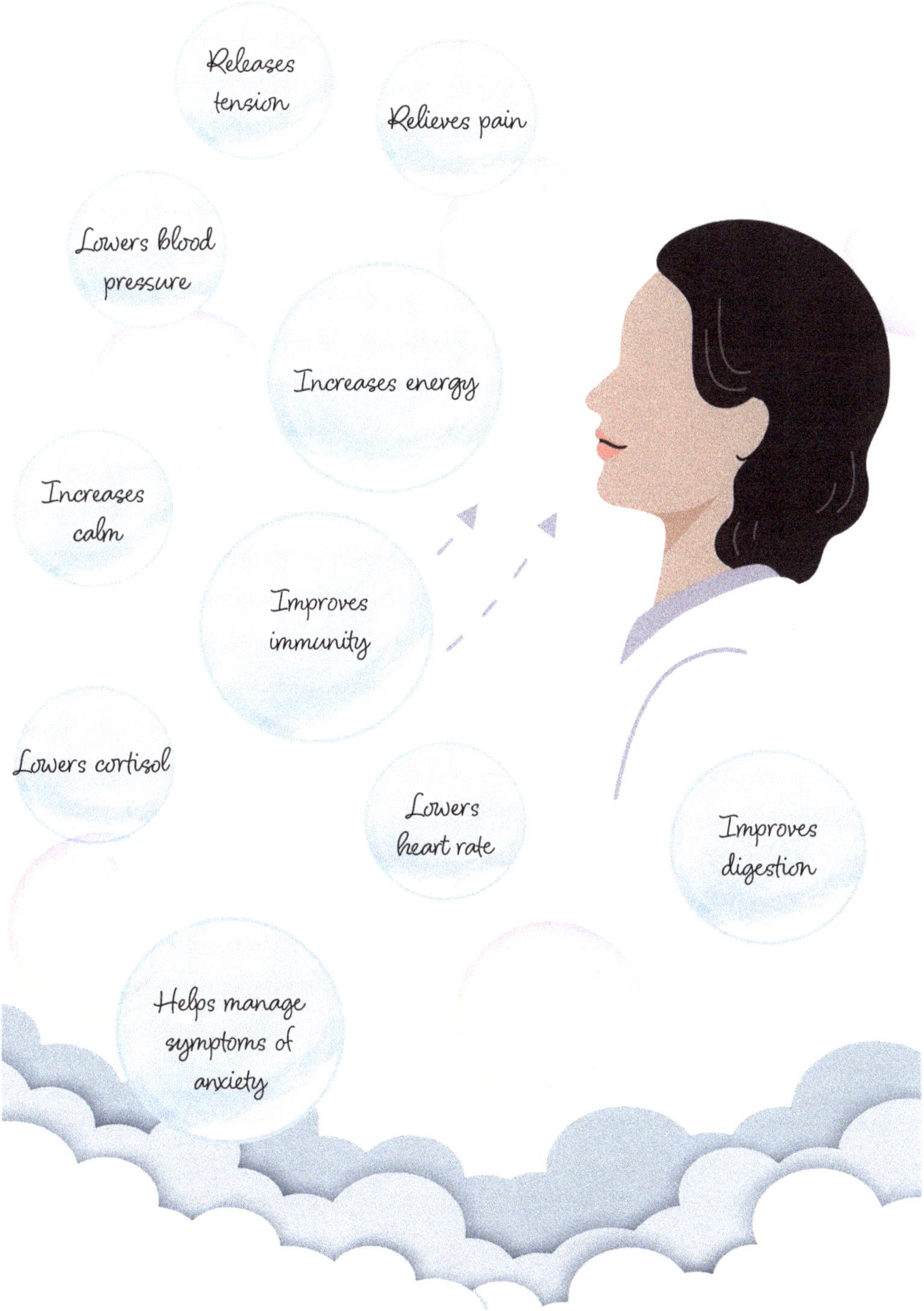

Deep Breathing

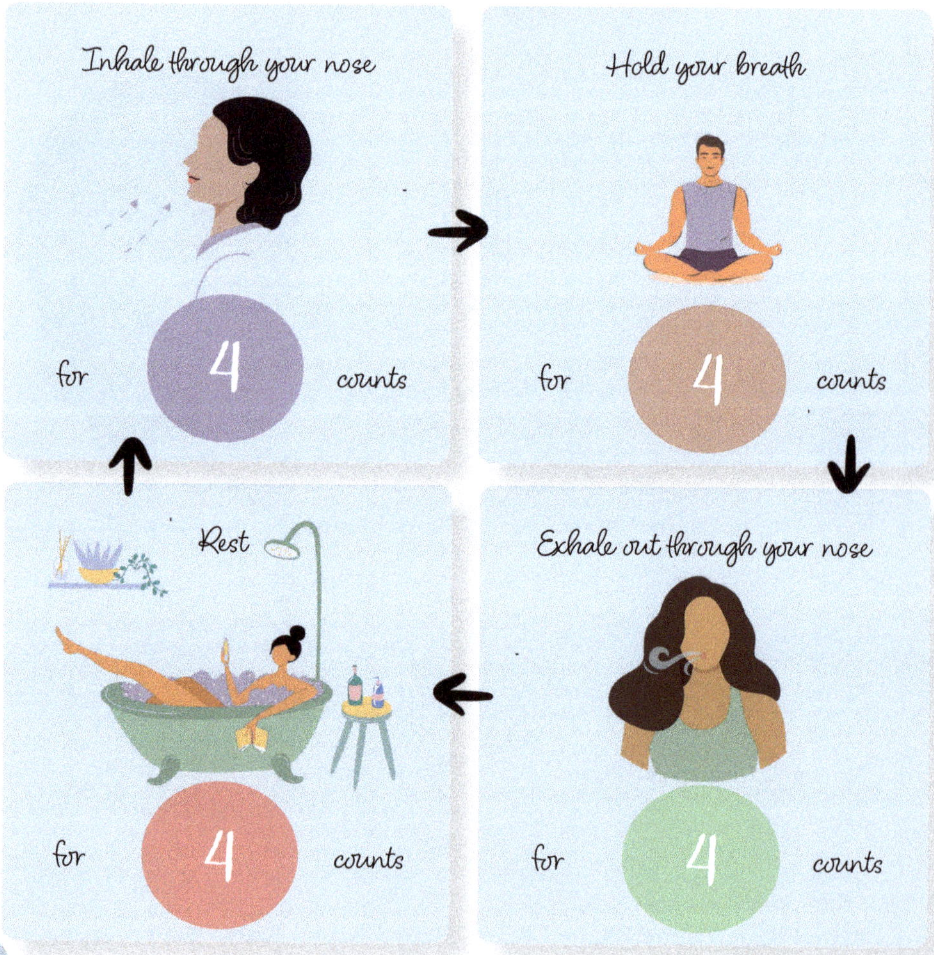

Six Types of Rest

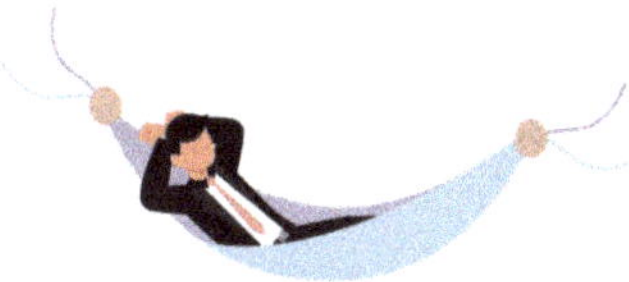

Physical

- maps
- breaks
- relaxation

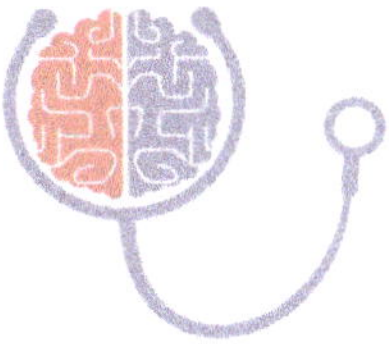

Mental

- meditation
- mindfulness
- music

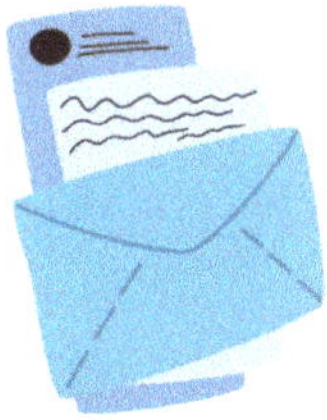

Creative

- coloring
- painting
- drawing

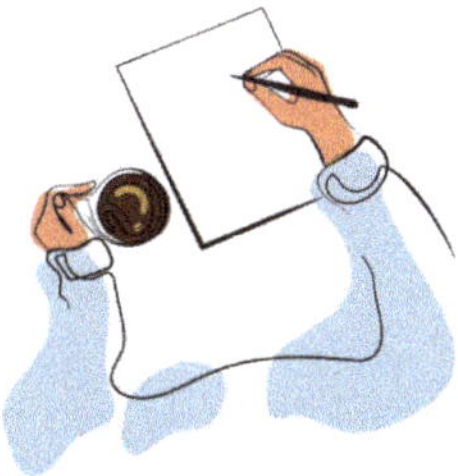

Spiritual

- journaling
- being in nature

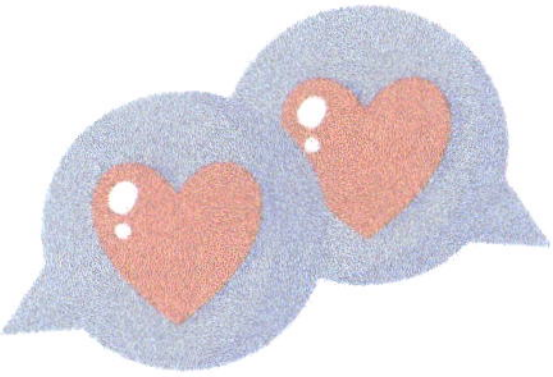

Emotional

- therapy
- talking to a friend

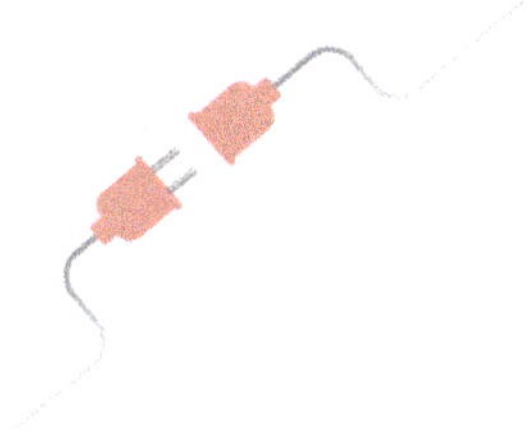

Sensory

- unplug from devices
- spending time alone

Are you looking for great ways to rest and relax? Consider incorporating rest from the following areas.

For each individual, rest can look very different, and what feels relaxing to me, may not be relaxing for you.

Therefore, it's important to figure out what makes you feel best and what recharges you physically and mentally.

Physical, mental, creative, spiritual, emotional, and sensory rest are all important to recharge and be your best self.

What are your favorite types of rest?
Note the categories below:

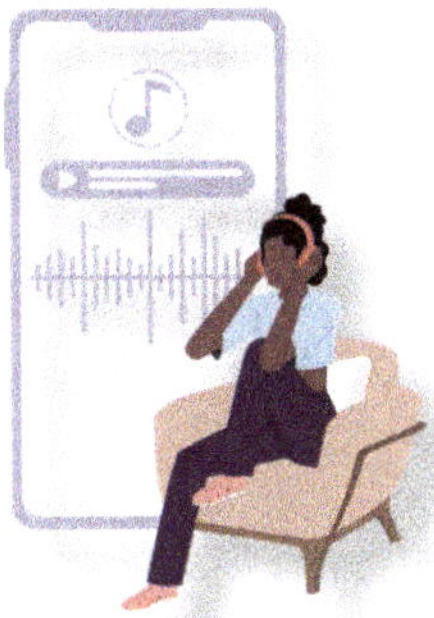

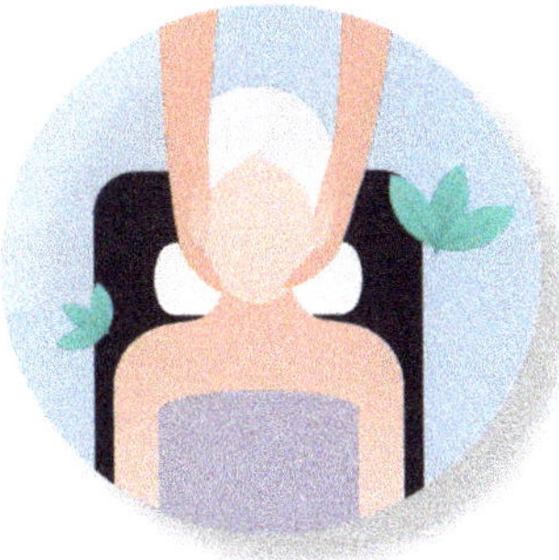

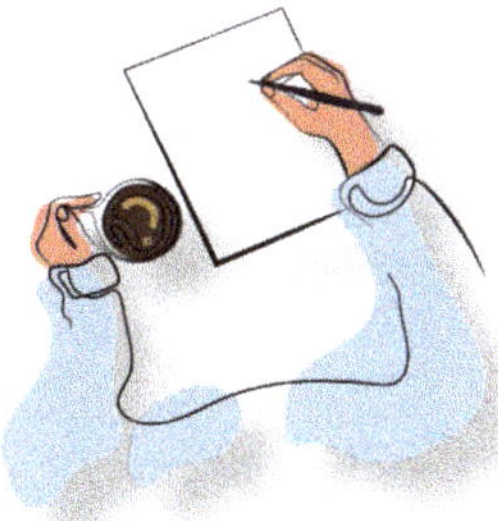

I will commit to getting more rest by ....

day 30

Ground Yourself

Grounding is eliminating all outside distractions and focusing only on our body and the present moment. When we practice grounding we pay close attention to our senses, our bodily sensations, and your surroundings. Grounding exercises are beneficial by distracting us from feelings of panic and worry; bringing us back to the present moment by focusing on our body and our surroundings. (p.333)

Weekend HAPPY

Things I should do when I feel tired:

Things I'm looking forward to:

Self Care For Exhaustion

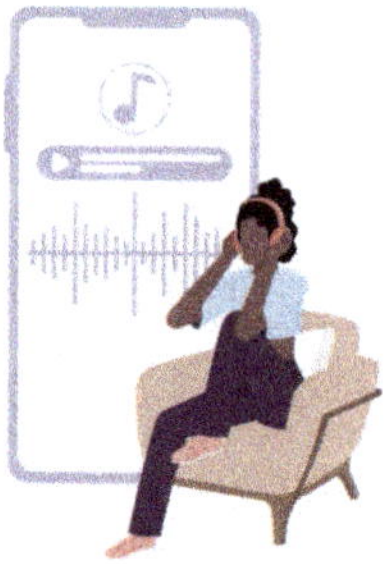

Listen to your favorite music playlist

Shhhhh....

Retreat to a quiet space

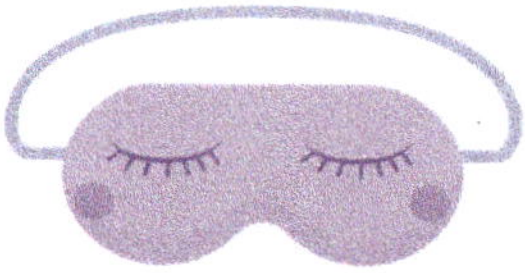

Go to sleep early

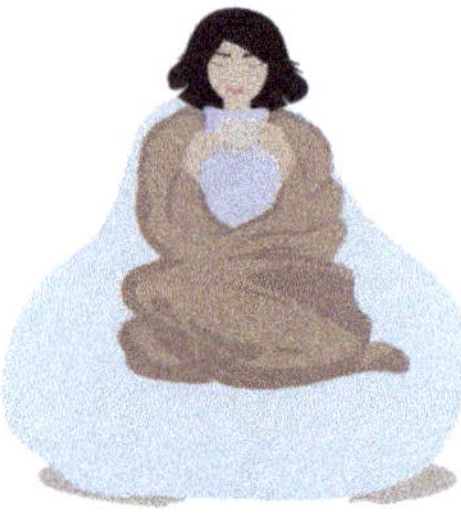

Curl up with a weighted blanket

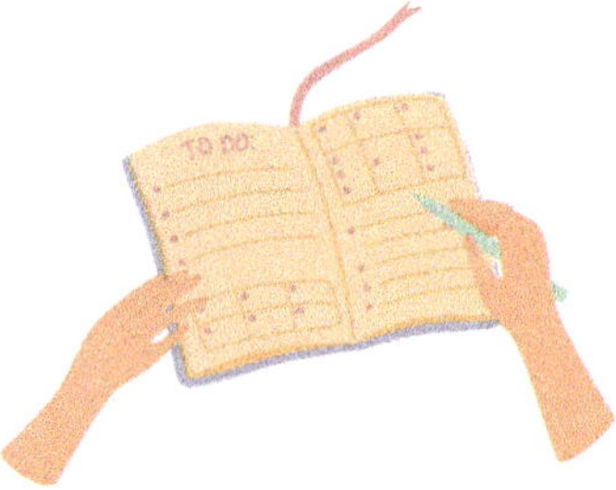

Make a list of high priority tasks

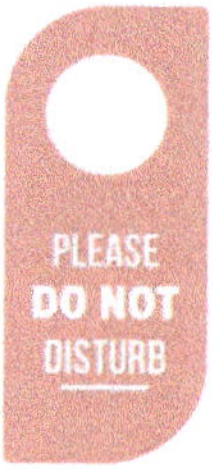

Turn your phone on do not disturb

Feeling burnt out or completely exhausted; why?

These tips are for you! Self care is a great way to recharge our bodies mentally and physically!

Our sleep quality directly impacts our mood, energy, and focus. Try getting 7-9 hours of sleep each night and removing all distractions at least 30 minutes before you plan to go to sleep.

Another way to reduce exhaustion is to curl up in comfy clothes with a weighted blanket once you are done with your daily responsibilities.

You can also put in headphones and jam out to your fav music playlist (p.159). Research shows that music can help reduce anxiety, and improve sleep quality, mood, alertness, and memory.

If your exhaustion tends to be accompanied by anxiety, It may be helpful for you to make a list of responsibilities. Separate priorities from tasks that can be completed at a later time, and focus only on completing the priorities now.

Ground Yourself in 10 Seconds

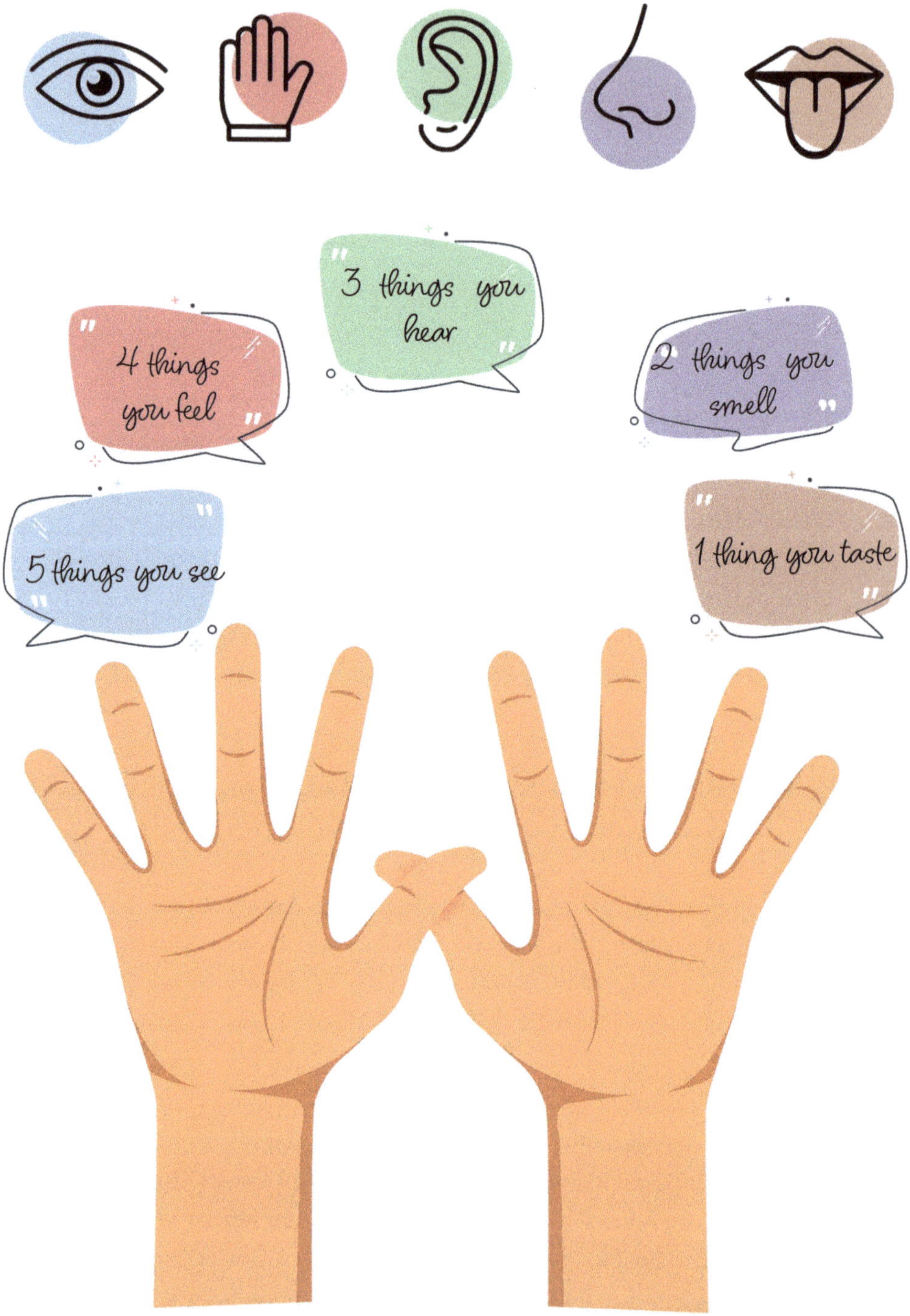

Get Grounded

After trying the grounding exercise,
what did you notice...

In your body?

Get Grounded

After trying the grounding exercise, what did you notice...

In your mind?

Get Grounded

After trying the grounding exercise,
what did you notice...

In your emotions (feelings)?

Get Grounded

After trying the grounding exercise, what did you notice...

In your space?

Compliment Yourself

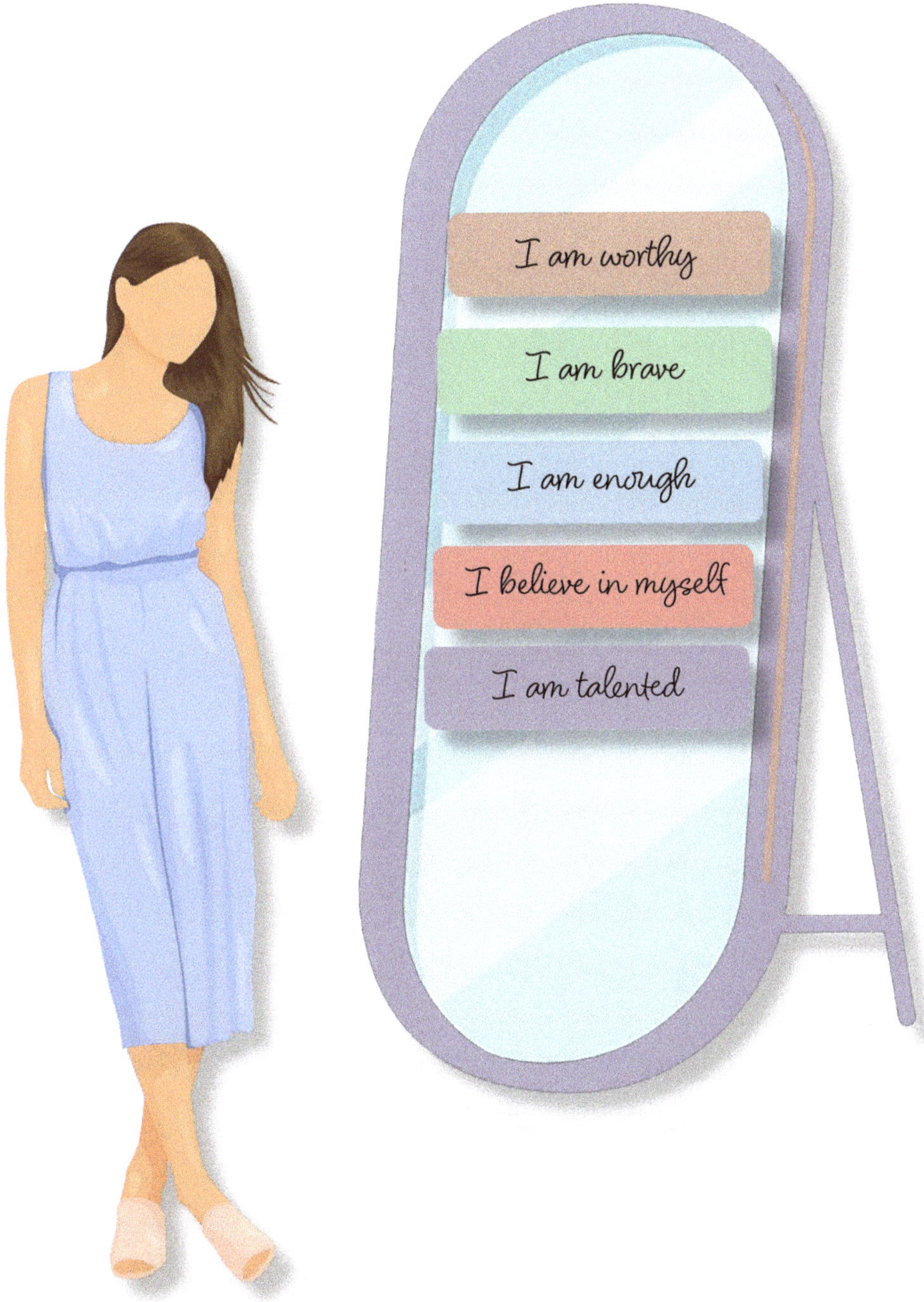

How will I compliment myself more and what will I say to me?

YAY ME Bingo

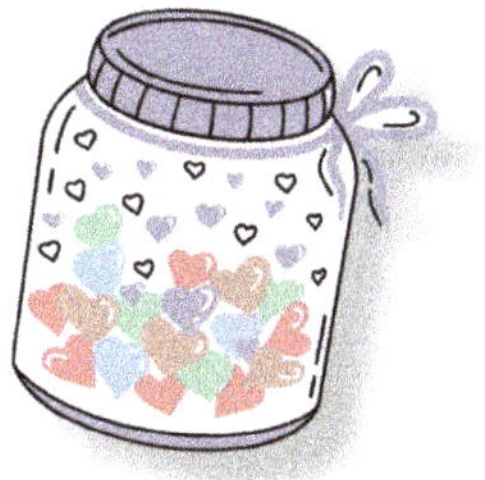

Offered to help someone	Baked some treats	Allowed myself to rest	Enjoyed time with friends and family
Forgave someone	Smiled at others	Lended out something	Made a new friend
Wrote myself a kind note	Spent time outside	Tried something new	Cleaned up my space
Did something that brought me joy	Brightened someone's day	Complimented someone	Did chores

day 31

Create Your Vision Board

Holistic Wellness Strategies aim to help individuals achieve balance and integration in their lives, by addressing all aspects of their being such as career, relationships, health, personal growth, fun, finances, family, and growth. It can include a range of techniques and interventions, such as mindfulness meditation, yoga, nutrition, and exercise to help target and improve overall well-being.

(p.334)

How can you increase your holistic mindfulness everyday? Write down one goal for each area.

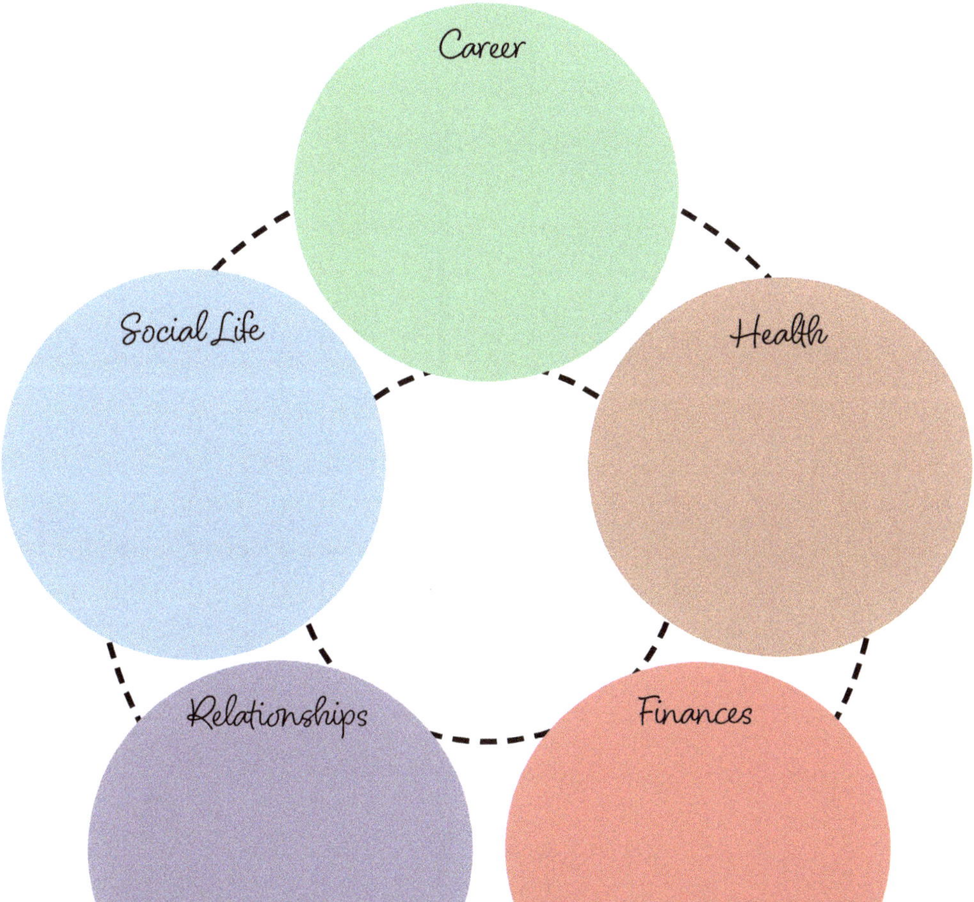

Ways To Boost Your Mind, Body, and Spirit

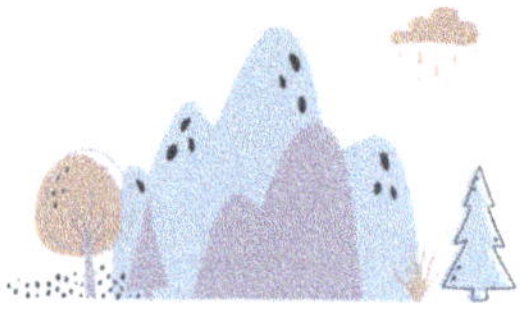

Spending time in fresh air

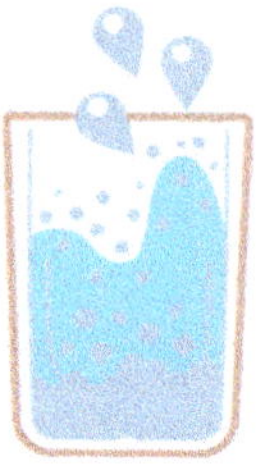

Drinking 2 liters of water

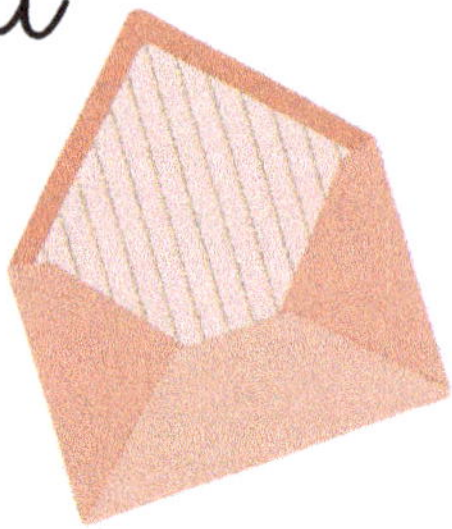

Writing yourself a kind letter

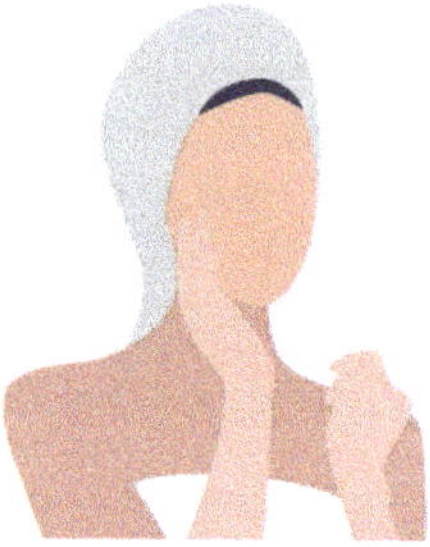

Creating a morning routine

Decluttering your room

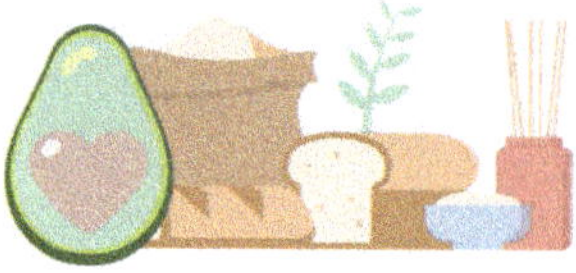

Making a healthy meal

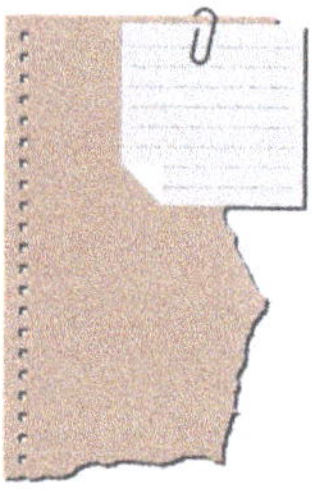

Making a list of daily gratitudes

Learning something new

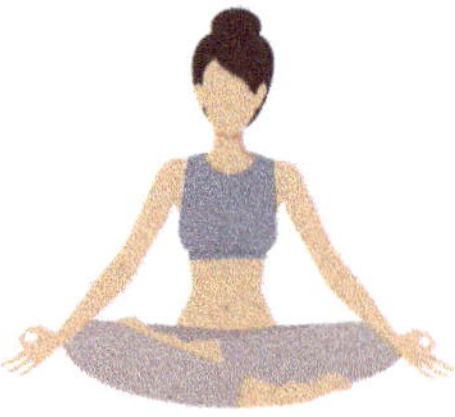

Yoga and meditation

The effects of stress and trauma go beyond the mind. They negatively impact the body and spirit as well.

Those who experience more adversities during childhood are increasingly likely to suffer from physical ailments in their adult lives, and to have more negative health outcomes due to the increased stress and trauma they've experienced.

However, there are ways to activate healing and to begin to work through trauma and stress.

You can do this by engaging in self-care that boosts all three areas of your health such as practicing yoga, meditation, spending time outside, and creating a routine.

By incorporating just a few of these activities daily, you can moderate the effects of unpleasant reminders or stressors, and navigate personal growth.

How are you going to boost your mind, body, and soul today?

DIY Vision Board

A vision is meant to inspire you and help you cultivate your dreams! Your vision board can include anything and everything that inspires you; no matter how big or small. This can consist of many things such as pictures, favorite quotes, memories/memorabilia, postcards, and words. Divide your vision board into 8 equal parts:

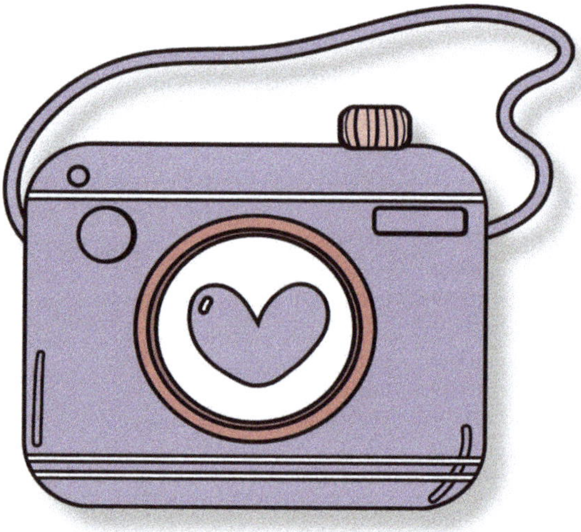

- Relationships
- Romance
- Home
- Career
- Vacation
- Mind
- Body
- Spirit

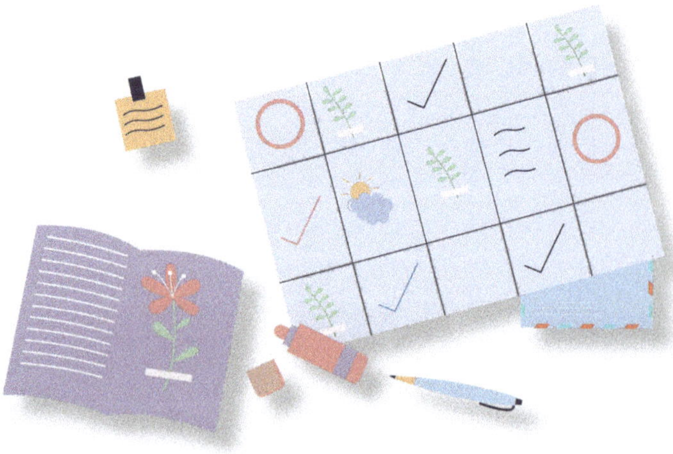

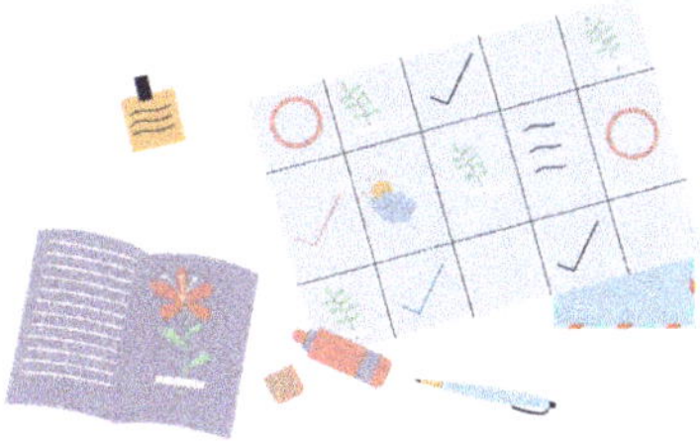

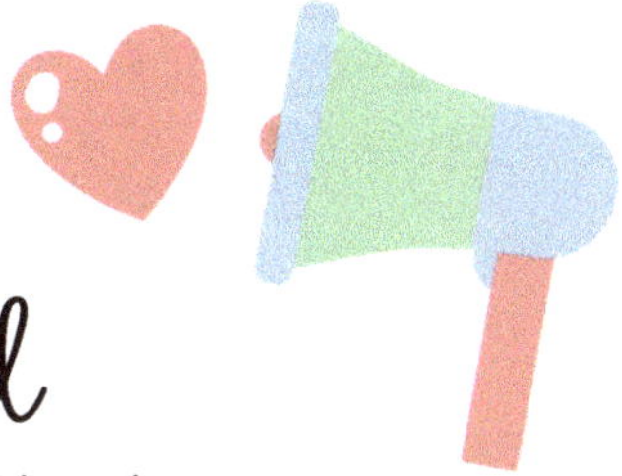

Vision Board

Write your wishes below in the boxes

Career

Finances

Relationships

Family

Personal Growth

Health

Fun

Growth

Weekly Review

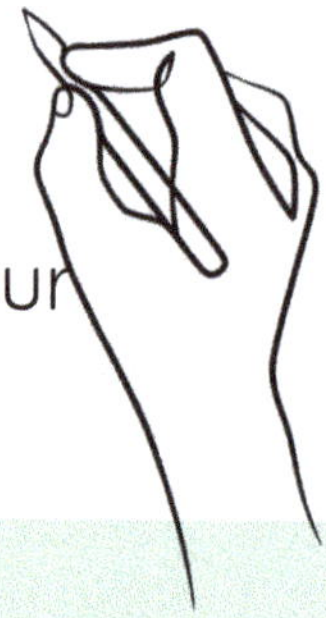

Take a moment to reflect on your progress and growth...

What have you been focusing on this week?	
What actions have you taken this week?	
What accomplishments have you had	
What challenges did you face?	
What limiting beliefs have you let go of?	

"Everything has its wonders, even darkness and silence, and I learn, whatever state I may be in, therein to be content."

Helen Keller

Wrapping Up Extras

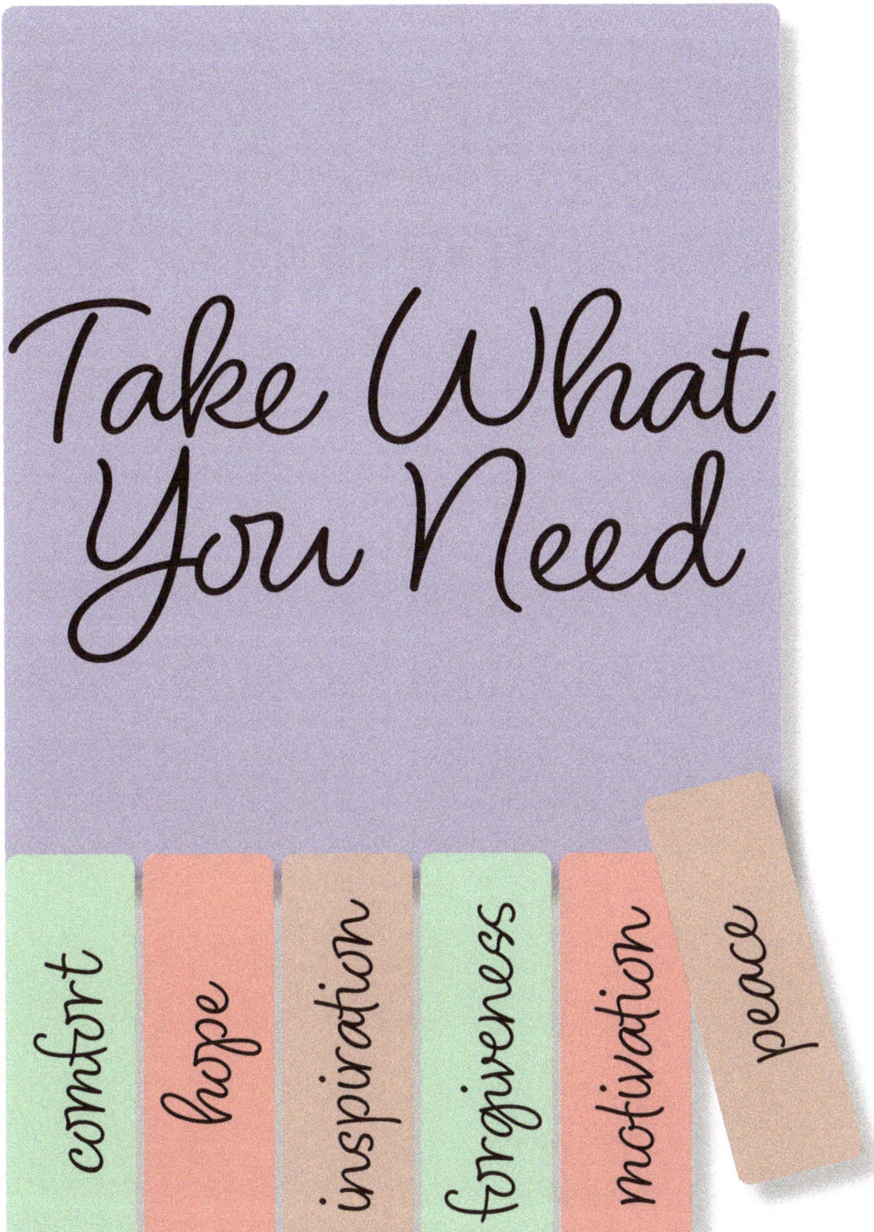
Take What You Need
comfort
hope
inspiration
forgiveness
motivation
peace

Signs That You Are HEALING

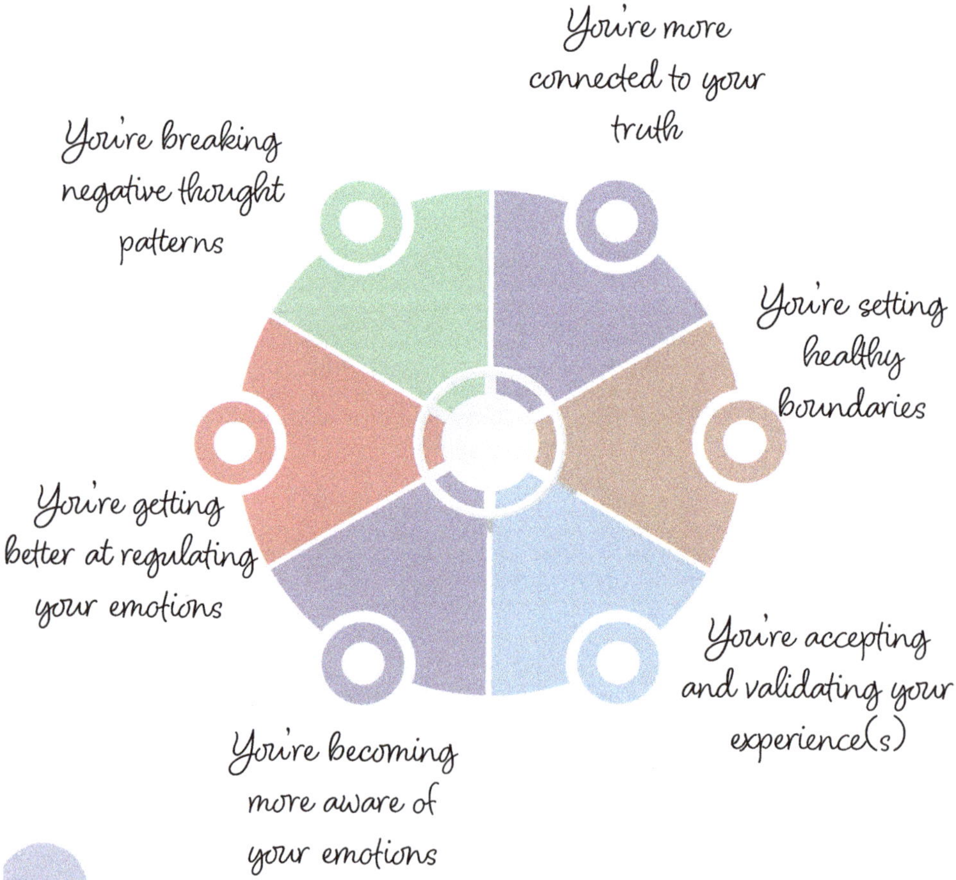

Your Playbook

Design a play by play book for your top 3 skills that help you with emotional regulation.

Some ideas to choose from:

4x4 breathing (p.297)

thought stopping (p.55)

self care activities (p.303)

self love mantra (p.70)

get up & move (p.114)

Write the skill and play by play instructions - keep it with you so when you need a reminder, it's always there. My personal therapy hack - sticky notes and index cards! Which 3 Skills are you going to commit to for next month:

The NEXT 30-DAY Self Care Challenge

Write a letter	Go for a walk	Practice yoga	Light a candle	Take a nap
Go to bed earlier	Write a bucket list	Eat healthy food	Watch your fav movie	Play
Pamper yourself	Go on a solo date	Practice gratitude	Try a DIY project	Ask for a hug
Explore a new part of your city	Spend time in nature	Write in a journal	Read a book	Watch the sunrise
Sit in the sun	Start a new hobby	Spa day at home	Grow a plant	Watch the sunset
Eat mindfully	Learn a new skill	Set small goals	Drink plenty of water	Call a friend

In Case You Forgot...

All you can do is stay true to you

"Remember to give yourself grace"

You are never a burden

You have always been enough

HELLO
my name is
You are valued

It's okay to rest when you need to

"You are allowed to take up space"

Conclusion

Congratulations! You completed 31 days of self-care with Give Yourself Self Love: A Journal for Non-Journalers! This is a fantastic achievement; celebrate your hard work! You've chosen yourself each day and made time for self-growth and self-improvement. As you tapped into micro self-care, used evidence-based skills, and developed a daily skills routine, you've grown closer to living your best life! Over 31 days, you've likely identified areas of change, challenged negative thoughts and beliefs, and gained new perspectives about yourself. Continue to revisit the daily key terms to help remind you of important ideas, concepts and skills that you've learned. Remember to put them on sticky notes to help jog your memory and increase your emotional stamina. Emotional stamina is the capacity to handle and cope with challenging or stressful situations involving the ability to maintain a sense of emotional balance, resilience, and well-being. You took the leap and decided to do something for yourself. A final 5 questions to ask yourself:

1. How did it work out?
2. How did it make you feel?
3. In what ways have you gotten to know yourself better?
4. What are you going to commit to continue your growth action plan?
5. What will you do to love yourself more every day?

When you started this journey you may have been unsure how little daily changes would help; and if you would notice any changes. Through practicing positive strategies from over the last 31 days you have subconsciously begun to rewire your brain to create more positive thought patterns. This is powerful work; you are in control of your thinking creating the life you love! I hope this process has encouraged you. By picking up this workbook and working through Give Yourself Self Love: A Journal for Non-Journaler, you have invested in yourself, and taken the time to reflect and grow. As you continue your self-care journey, a gentle reminder to celebrate YOU: the amazing self-love changes that you are capable of achieving.

By continuing to improve and redevelop your personal growth action plan, you'll continue to learn how to overcome challenges, develop your new skills, and cultivate your new sense of self facilitating change; continue to go back through the workbook and revisit the pages that are particularly useful for you. Using Give Yourself Self Love: A Journal for Non-Journalers, repetitively you will continue to solidify your growth mindset while expanding your knowledge, self-love skills, self-love discovery: now you are thriving instead of surviving! So, my challenge for you is that you continue to pinpoint what brings you joy; and, how you can incorporate more joy into your daily self-care practice.

Glossary

Accountability refers to the responsibility and answerability for one's actions or decisions. It involves being willing to take ownership of the consequences of one's behavior and to accept the consequences of one's actions; which, involves being reliable, trustworthy, and transparent in one's dealings with others. Being accountable is willing to admit mistakes and take corrective action.

Action refers to the process of doing something to achieve a desired outcome or goal. Action involves taking steps towards a specific objective and can be either physical or mental in nature. Actions can be small, such as making a phone call, or larger, such as launching a new business venture. Taking action is important for achieving success and making progress towards one's goals.

Anxiety is a normal emotion that is characterized by feelings of worry, fear, apprehension, and/or somatic symptoms associated with future events or uncertain situations.[1] It is a natural response to internal or external stress or danger, and can be adaptive in certain situations, such as preparing for a job interview or exam.[2] However, when anxiety becomes excessive, persistent, or interferes with daily functioning, it can be considered a disorder.

Appreciation refers to the act of recognizing and valuing the worth or importance of something or someone. It can be shown in various ways such as expressing gratitude, admiration, or respect towards someone or for something. Appreciation can also refer to an increase in the value of an asset over time, such as a stock or a piece of real estate.

Attachment, in psychology, refers to the emotional bond that develops between an infant and their primary caregiver. It is a critical aspect of social and emotional development,

1 American Psychiatric Association. (2013). Glossary of Technical Terms. Diagnostic and statistical manual of mental disorders (5th ed.).
2 APA. (2013). Diagnostic and statistical manual (5th ed.).

and it has been extensively studied by psychologists and researchers.

Attunement refers to the ability to be fully present and emotionally responsive to another person's needs and feelings. It involves being able to tune in and empathize with another person's emotional state and respond in a way that is supportive and helpful. Attunement is an important aspect of healthy relationships, particularly in parent-child relationships and therapeutic relationships.

Authenticity refers to the quality of being genuine, honest, and true to oneself. It involves expressing oneself in a way that is consistent with one's values, beliefs, and personality, rather than conforming to social norms or expectations. Authenticity involves being self-aware, introspective, and reflective, and being willing to take risks and be vulnerable. It is a process of self-discovery and self-expression, where individuals strive to align their outer behavior with their inner feelings and desires.

Beliefs are thoughts and feelings that we believe to be true or accept to be true about yourself regardless of evidence or fact. Our beliefs can come from our upbringing, past experiences, social interactions, education, culture, societal norms and relationships. The beliefs that we hold often inform our actions, decision-making, feelings and behaviors that we value impacting the way we think.

Blame iis the act of holding someone responsible for a fault or wrongdoing; an attribution of responsibility for a negative outcome or situation. Blame can be directed towards oneself or others, and it can be harmful depending on the situation. In some cases, blame can be a helpful way of holding people accountable for their actions and encouraging them to take responsibility for their mistakes. And, allowing us to set healthy boundaries for ourselves.

Body Positivity is a philosophy that promotes the acceptance and celebration of all bodies, regardless of their size, shape, or or appearance; encouraging individuals to embrace their bodies as they are. Body positivity involves promoting self-love, self-care, and self-acceptance, and rejecting the idea that there is one "ideal" body type or shape.

Boundaries refer to the limits or guidelines that individuals set for themselves in response to others about what is acceptable behavior or treatment when in relationships. Boundaries can be physical, emotional, mental, intimate, professional or spiritual, and can vary depending on the individual and the situation. For example, physical boundaries may involve personal space, privacy, or touch, while emotional boundaries may involve expressing one's feelings, needs, or opinions.

Character Traits are our unique individual qualities or attributes that make us who we are. Many of us have unique qualities that impact our personality and how we relate to others. It's important to identify your unique thoughts and behaviors as well as how they can be your "superpowers" within your life. Through selecting our favorite internal qualities we can better understand and celebrate ourselves.

Connection is a sense of belonging and closeness which consists of the various relationships to others, experiences, thoughts, emotions and behaviors that we form throughout lives. Our interconnectedness to ourselves and others allows us to feel fulfilled and loved. Having a strong connection with yourself is important to acknowledge and validate our feelings, thoughts, expectations, beliefs, and attitudes.

Coping is the ability to develop strategies that help us to manage stressful or potentially harmful situations. Healthy coping strategies, such as going for a walk, tapping, listening to music, and lowering stress can help us to reduce the impact of stressful situations by making them more manageable.

Core Beliefs are the deeply held beliefs developed early in life and shaped by our personal experiences, culture, values, spirituality and upbringing that affects what we believe about ourselves, others, and the world. Core beliefs impact our self-confidence and deeply impact how we feel about ourselves in relationship to others. When we shift these beliefs to be more positive and realistic, it allows us to develop new perspectives on life; creating more connection to the world around us.

Empathy is the ability to comprehend and appreciate others' experiences and feelings.[3] It involves being able to see things from another person's perspective, and to feel and respond to their emotions in a compassionate and supportive way. Empathy is an important aspect of social and emotional intelligence, as it allows individuals to connect with others on an emotional level, build relationships, and navigate social situations effectively.

Emotional Adversity is the ability to overcome rigidity, fear, stuck points, and pain by moving into emotionally intelligent behavior. By learning to manage our emotions through regulation and skill development, we can open our minds to growth promoting change and cultivating a present, calm, mindset.

Emotional Attunement is when you are aware in addition to being responsive to others' needs. This is a fundamentally important skill in interpersonal, romantic and professional relationships. When you're emotionally attuned to others, you're responsive, open, understanding and supportive of the other person's emotional state. Emotional attunement doesn't mean that you are responsible for other people's emotional state; rather, you're responsive to their emotional needs.

Emotional Intelligence refers to the ability to recognize, understand, and regulate one's own emotions, as well as the emotions of others. It involves being able to identify and manage one's own emotions, as well as being able to empathize with and understand the emotions of others. Emotional intelligence can be divided into several different components, including: self awareness, self-regulation, motivation, empathy, and social skills.

3, American Psychiatric Association. (2013). Glossary of Technical Terms. Diagnostic and statistical manual of mental disorders (5th ed.).

Emotional Regulation refers to the ability to manage and regulate your own emotions in a healthy and effective way. It involves being able to recognize and understand your emotions, as well as being able to control and modify them in response to different situations. Emotional regulation can involve several different strategies, including: self-soothing, cognitive reappraisal, problem-solving, seeking support.

Feelings are subjective experiences that arise from our emotions, thoughts, and physical sensations. They can be positive or negative, ranging from subtle to overwhelming. Common feelings include happiness, sadness, anger, fear, joy, love, and contentment. Feelings can influence our behavior, decisions, and overall well-being.

Goals are the desired outcomes or achievements that a person wants to attain. They help provide direction and motivation, which can be either short-term or long-term in nature. Setting goals can be helpful in personal and professional development, by clarifying what is important as well as needed to be accomplished.

Gratitude refers to a feeling of appreciation, thankfulness, or recognition for the good things in one's life. It involves acknowledging and being mindful of the positive aspects of one's experiences, relationships, and circumstances, rather than focusing on the negative or lacking aspects. Gratitude can be directed towards oneself, others, or a higher power or source.

Grounding is eliminating all outside distractions and focusing only on our body and the present moment. When we practice grounding we pay close attention to our senses, our bodily sensations, and your surroundings. Grounding exercises are beneficial by distracting us from feelings of panic and worry; bringing us back to the present moment by focusing on our body and our surroundings.

Happiness is a positive emotional state characterized by feelings of contentment, satisfaction,and pleasure. It is often associated with joy, fulfillment, and a sense of well-being. Happiness can be experienced in response to various stimuli, such as achieving a goal, spending time with loved ones, engaging in activities we enjoy, or simply appreciating the beauty of the world around us.

Holistic Wellness Strategies aim to help individuals achieve balance and integration in their lives, by addressing all aspects of their being such as career, relationships, health, personal growth, fun, finances, family, and growth. It can include a range of techniques and interventions, such as mindfulness meditation, yoga, nutrition, and exercise to help target and improve overall well-being.

Joy is our level of happiness or satisfaction within our daily lives. Joy, the emotion of happiness, is often evoked by good well-being and is the result of something positive happening to us. Although we derive joy from successes and good events, we can also create our own joy and happiness through our daily intentions and actions.

Meditation is a mental exercise that involves training the brain by focusing the mind on a specific object, thought, or activity, in order to achieve a state of deep relaxation and concentration. Meditation can be practiced in many different ways, such as through mindfulness meditation, transcendental meditation, or loving-kindness meditation.

Mindfulness is a practice that involves being fully present and engaged in the present moment, without judgment or distraction. It involves paying attention to your thoughts, feelings, and bodily sensations, and observing them with curiosity and openness. Mindfulness can be practiced through a variety of techniques, such as meditation, breathing exercises, or simply paying attention to your surroundings.

Perfectionism is a personality trait characterized by the tendency to set extremely high standards for oneself and others, while striving for flawlessness and excellence in all areas of life. Perfectionists often have a strong need for control, and may be highly critical of themselves and others when those standards are not met. Perfectionism can become problematic when it leads to unrealistic expectations, excessive self-criticism, and the belief that things can only be done a certain way.[4]

Positive Self-talk is speaking to ourselves in a way that is uplifting and kind. Positive self-talk involves offering validation and compassion to ourselves. Although we may experience difficult times, positive self-talk is a great way to avoid getting stuck in negative thought patterns and to instead invest in our well-being by cultivating self-love.

Self-care refers to activities and practices that individuals engage in to promote their physical, mental, emotional and spiritual well-being. Self-care can be an important component of maintaining overall health and preventing stress which can cause burnout. Self-Care activities include: physical self-care, emotional self-care, mental self-care, social self-care, and spiritual self-care.

Self-esteem refers to an individual's overall subjective evaluation of their worth, value, and adequacy as a person; to the degree at which they see themselves as capable, lovable, and deserving of respect and dignity. Self-esteem can be influenced by a range of factors, including one's upbringing, experiences, achievements, and social relationships.

Self-love refers to the practice of caring for, accepting, and valuing oneself. It involves developing a positive and nurturing relationship with oneself, recognizing one's worth, and prioritizing one's own well-being. Self-love encompasses self-compassion, self-acceptance, and maintaining healthy boundaries. It is an essential aspect of personal growth, contributing to improved mental, emotional, and physical well-being.

4 American Psychiatric Association. (2013). Glossary of Technical Terms. Diagnostic and statistical manual of mental disorders (5th ed.).

Shame is an intense feeling of embarrassment, humiliation, or disgrace that arises when a person believes they have failed to meet certain social standards or expectations- what we believe about how we are perceived in the world. It can result from a sense of inadequacy, failure, or wrong-doing, and can be accompanied by feelings of guilt or self-blame.

Stress Management consists of strategies that help to manage stress on a day to day basis over time. When we are feeling stressed out, these strategies and coping skills can help us to reduce our stressors by establishing a sense of calm, stimulate relaxation and improve mood.

Values are the beliefs, principles, and ideals that are important to you. They are the fundamental concepts and standards that guide your behavior, decision-making, and interactions with others. Values can be influenced by a variety of factors, such as culture, religion, personal experiences, and social conditioning.

"What" Questions allow you to move towards something, keeping you present-focused and able to move into solutions thus finding resolutions. What questions can help you make an action plan to stop anxiety or the fear of the unknown; allowing you to modify and change unwanted behavior patterns and create new habits.

"Why" Questions allow you to move into processing by analyzing the past. Why questions are important to help you discover your past thoughts, feelings, behaviors and where you're getting stuck, by examining your core beliefs. By analyzing your past, you can identify those behaviors that aren't serving you anymore and move into new ways of behaving, thinking, and being.

References

American Psychological Association. (2021). The Road to Resilience. *University of North Carolina Wilmington.* June, 20, 2021.
https://uncw.edu/studentaffairs/committees/pdc/documents/the%20road%20to%20resilience.pdf

American Psychiatric Association. (2013). Glossary of Technical Terms. *Diagnostic and statistical manual of mental disorders* (5th ed.).

Bishop, G. J. (2016). *Unfu*k Yourself: Get Out of Your Head and into Your Life.* CreateSpace Independent Publishing Platform.

Bonham-Carter, D. (2012). *Introducing Self-Esteem: A Practical Guide.* Icon.

Burns, D. D. (2012). *Feeling Good: The New Mood Therapy.* HarperCollins.

Carson, R. (2009). A Master Class in Gremlin-Taming: T*he Absolutely Indispensable Next Step for Freeing Yourself from the Monster of the Mind.* HarperCollins.

Duhigg, C. (2012). *The Power of Habit: Why We Do What We do in Life and Business.* Random House Publishing Group.

Dweck, C. S. (2007). Mindset: *The New Psychology.* Random House Publishing Group.

Harris, D. (2017). 10% Happier: *How I Tamed the Voice in My Head, Reduced Stress Without Losing My Edge, and Found Self-Help That Actually Works - A True Story.* Hodder & Stoughton.

Joseph, S. (2012). *What Doesn't Kill Us The New Psychology of Posttraumatic Growth.* Little Brown Book Group.

Kabat-Zinn, J. (2013). *Full Catastrophe Living (Revised Edition): Using the Wisdom of Your Body and Mind to Face Stress, Pain, and Illness.* Random House Publishing Group.

Kallos-Lilly, V., & Fitzgerald, J. (2014). An Emotionally Focused Workbook for Couples: The Two of Us. Taylor & Francis.

Knipe, J. (2014). *EMDR Toolbox: Theory and Treatment of Complex PTSD and Dissociation.* Springer Publishing Company.

Linehan, M. M. (2015). D*BT Skills Training Handouts and Worksheets, Second Edition.* Guildford Publications.

McKay, M., & Sutker, C. (2009). *The Self-Esteem Guided Journal.* ReadHowYouWant.

McKay, M., Wood, J. C., & Brantley, J. (2019). *The Dialectical Behavior Therapy Skills Workbook: Practical DBT Exercises for Learning Mindfulness, Interpersonal Effectiveness, Emotion Regulation, and Distress Tolerance.* New Harbinger Publications.

Porges, S. W. (2017).*The Pocket Guide To The Polyvagal Theory: The Transformative Power of Feeling Safe.* W. W. Norton.

Poulter, S. B. (2019). *The Shame Factor: Heal Your Deepest Fears and Set Yourself Free.* Prometheus Books.

Rendon, J. (2015). *Upside: The New Science of Post-Traumatic Growth.* Touchstone.

Resick, P. A., Monson, C. M., & Chard, K. M. (2016). C*ognitive Processing Therapy for PTSD: A Comprehensive Manual.* Guilford Publications.

Rossy, L. (2016). *The Mindfulness-Based Eating Solution: Proven Strategies to End Overeating, Satisfy Your Hunger, and Savor Your Life.* New Harbinger Publications.

Sarno, J. E. (2009). T*he Divided Mind: The Epidemic of Mind-body Disorders.* HarperCollins.

Tedeschi, R. G., & Moore, B. A. (2016). *The Posttraumatic Growth Workbook: Coming Through Trauma Wiser, Stronger, and More Resilient.* New Harbinger Publications.

Tedeschi, R., Moore, B., Falke, K., & Goldberg J. (2020). *Transformed By Trauma: Stories of Posttrauamatic Growth.* Independently Published.

Tedeschi, R, G., Shakespeare-Finch, J., Taku, K., & Calhoun, L. G. (2018). *Posttraumatic Growth: Theory, Research, and Applications.* Taylor & Francis.

Van der Kolk, B. A. (2015). *The Body Keeps The Score.* Penguin Publishing Group.

Joelle is a highly acclaimed international speaker, licensed psychotherapist, and trauma expert with a global following. Joelle holds a Masters of Arts degree in Education, a Masters of Fine Arts degree in Dance, a Masters of Counseling Psychology with a specialization in Trauma Degree, and clinical PhD of Psychology with dissertation candidate. She is also the author of a TED-Ed video on PTSD that has garnered over 3.2 million views and is available in 28 different languages. Joelle has been featured as a guest on numerous podcasts and has been recognized as a top executive coach and mentor. Her focus is on helping people overcome obstacles and lead fulfilling, balanced lives. In addition, Joelle is a successful entrepreneur who coaches other business owners on how to follow their passions and create successful businesses. Joelle started JRM&A Inc. to help others discover their hopes, dreams and abilities to thrive through adversity, trauma and mental challenges. Her achievements include being a guest speaker on ABC's 60 Minutes: Beyond the Headlines, hosting Switch YouTube Live, and receiving the DOD's HIRE Vets Medallion Award and several Outstanding Achievement Awards for Top Female Executive. She is also about to launch a new series of therapy workbooks.

www.joellerabowmaletis.com

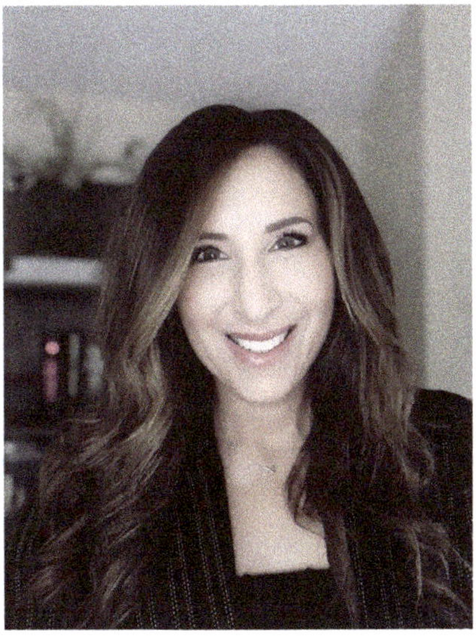

Acknowledgments

A million thank you's to Sarah Lucha, my right-hand woman, venting partner, fashionista stylist guru, and partner-in-shenanigans! Every day, you make it worth doing. Thank you for standing by me through thick and thin while we continue to grow Joelle Rabow Maletis & Associates, Inc (JRM&A).

Thank you to my psychological research assistant, Alyssa Bombacino, who has spent countless hours helping fine-tune empirically-based, user-friendly, and psychologically appropriate content for this self-help journal.

Jenny Ernest, JRM&A Senior Marketing Coordinator, your dedication and commitment are priceless. Thank you for providing a fresh perspective to this project and supporting the marketing efforts to let the world know about our contributions to providing wellness for all.

The JRM&A Team who have helped inspire the creation of this book: you are celebrated, appreciated, and honored as you have continued to help my vision of mental wellness grow.

A heartfelt thank you to my parents, publicist Lyda Mclallen, graphic designer Mattea Henderson, and my dear family and friends who have spent time reviewing pages - I appreciate each and every one of you!